Empowerment, Health Promotion and Young People

Globally, young people's health is an increasing priority area for health practitioners, policy-makers and researchers, and concepts of empowerment feature strongly in international public health discourses on young people's health. Yet the concept of empowerment remains under-theorized, and its relationship to young people's health is not well understood. This innovative volume critically examines the concept of empowerment and its relationship to young people's health.

Empowerment, Health Promotion and Young People is set out in two main parts. Part one examines differing conceptions of power and empowerment and how these concepts have been variously defined and used in relation to young people's health and health promotion. Part two offers a new theoretical framework for understanding empowerment as it relates to young people's health. Drawing together key works in the field and findings from an empirical enquiry on young people's health, this framework looks at health as it is defined by young people themselves, and offers new directions for empowerment, and critical insights into the field of young people's health and health promotion.

Critically engaging with the concept of power and opening up the debate about the relevance and effectiveness of using contemporary understandings of empowerment to promote health, this book is suitable for researchers and students of health, sociology, education and youth studies interested in young people's health and health promotion.

Grace Spencer is a Lecturer in Health at the School of Nursing, Midwifery & Physiotherapy at the University of Nottingham, UK.

Routledge Studies in Public Health

Available titles include:

Planning in Health Promotion Work
Roar Amdam

Alcohol, Tobacco and Obesity
Morality, Mortality and the New Public Health
Edited by Kirsten Bell, Amy Salmon and Darlene McNaughton

Population Mental Health
Evidence, Policy, and Public Health Practice
Edited by Neal Cohen and Sandro Galea

International Perspectives on Public Health and Palliative Care
Edited by Libby Sallnow, Suresh Kumar and Allan Kellehear

Organisational Capacity Building in Health Systems
Niyi Awofeso

Health and Health Promotion in Prisons
Michael Ross

Global Health Disputes and Disparities
A Critical Appraisal of International Law and Population Health
Dru Bhattacharya

Gender-Based Violence and Public Health
International Perspectives on Budgets and Policies
Edited by Keerty Nakray

Assembling Health Rights in Global Context
Genealogies and Anthropologies
Edited by Alex Mold and David Reubi

Empowerment, Health Promotion and Young People
A Critical Approach
Grace Spencer

Forthcoming titles:

Globalisation, Environmental Health and Social Justice
R. Scott Frey

Empowerment, Health Promotion and Young People

A Critical Approach

Grace Spencer

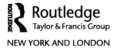
Routledge
Taylor & Francis Group

NEW YORK AND LONDON

First published 2014
by Routledge
2 Park Square, Milton Park, Abingdon, Oxon, OX14 4RN

and by Routledge
711 Third Avenue, New York, NY 10017

Routledge is an imprint of the Taylor & Francis Group, an informa business

© 2014 Grace Spencer

British Library Cataloguing-in-Publication Data
A catalogue record for this book is available from the British Library

Library of Congress Cataloging-in-Publication Data

Spencer, Grace, author.
  Empowerment, health promotion and young people : a critical approach / Grace Spencer.
    p. ; cm. — (Routledge studies in public health)
  I. Title. II. Series: Routledge studies in public health. [DNLM:
1. Health Promotion. 2. Adolescent. 3. Power (Psychology)
4. Young Adult. WA 590]
RA776
613—dc23   2013017694

ISBN13: 978-0-415-81040-1 (hbk)
ISBN13: 978-0-203-07103-8 (ebk)

Typeset in Sabon
by Apex CoVantage, LLC

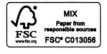

Printed and bound in Great Britain by
TJ International Ltd, Padstow, Cornwall

Contents

Tables and figures

Tables

Figure

Foreword

Understanding young people and health

How young people are viewed tells us a great deal about a society. Up until relatively recently in Europe, young people were viewed as little different from adults, being dressed in similar clothes to their elders and being expected to work and contribute to the household from a very early age (Ariès 1962). Such a view still prevails across much of Africa, Asia and Southern America, with boys and young men being expected to generate income outside the home whilst girls contribute to the domestic economy alongside their mothers and other female relatives.

Yet in the countries of Europe and especially in North America, images and understandings of youth have changed dramatically in the past 100 years. The impetus for much of the shift can be found in the writing of G. Stanley Hall, who earned the first psychology doctorate in the United States under William James at Harvard, who later taught psychology and pedagogy at Johns Hopkins University, and who then went on to become the first president of the American Psychological Association.

Hall's two-volume book, first published in 1904, entitled *Adolescence – Its Psychology and Its Relations to Physiology, Anthropology, Sociology, Sex, Crime, and Religion*, was very much a product of its time. A firm believer in eugenics, Hall was of the view that any charity toward those who were physically, emotionally or intellectually weak interfered with natural selection. Characterizing adolescence as a time of 'storm and stress', Hall saw this stage of life as one filled with mood disruptions, conflict with parents and risky behaviour. He wrote,

> The teens are emotionally unstable and pathic. It is a natural impulse to experience hot and perfervid psychic states, and it is characterized by emotionalism. We see here the instability and fluctuations now so characteristic. The emotions develop by contrast and reaction into the opposite. (Hall 1904, vol. 2, pp. 74–75)

As a writer on pedagogy, Hall believed that open discussion and critical opinions were not to be tolerated. Young people needed firm indoctrination to protect them from the individualism distorting the progress of U.S. culture. Instead, schools should induct their pupils into the selfless ideals of service, patriotism, body culture, military discipline, love of authority, awe of nature and devotion to the state (cited in Karrier 1986, p. 154).

Just over a century later, a quite different view was expressed by U.S. President Barack Obama in his second inaugural address. He said,

> America's possibilities are limitless, for we possess all the qualities that this world without boundaries demands: youth and drive; diversity and openness; an endless capacity for risk and a gift for reinvention. My fellow Americans, we are made for this moment, and we will seize it – so long as we seize it together. (cited in Curtis 2013)

Through its recognition of the value of risk taking and the potential derived from openness and change, Obama's speech signals a quite different perspective on youth and 'youthfulness', pointing to the potential for creativity, opportunity and progress. A similar kind of perspective underpinned the view of early 20th-century social reformers writing, somewhat paradoxically, around the same time as G. Stanley Hall. One of the most prominent of these, Jane Addams, argued forcefully for the power and potential of youth:

> We may either smother the divine fire in youth or we may feed it. We may either stand stupidly staring as it sinks into a murky fire of crime and flares into the intermittent blaze of folly, or we may tend it into a lambent flame with power to make clean and bright our dingy city streets. (Addams 1909, pp. 161–162)

In her book *The Spirit of Youth and the City Streets,* Addams (1909) stressed the importance of free speech, play and recreation in building on the spirit of youth. Hull House, a Chicago settlement house that she established with her partner Ellen Gates Starr in 1889 offered wide-ranging programmes in drama and art, boys' and girls' clubs, language classes, a free-speech atmosphere and a playground. Democratic cooperation and collective action were promoted, building on the spirit of young people to transform and change the world. Beyond the United States, young people's potential to effect change later came to be fêted across a wide and diverse range of contexts: in the Hitler youth movements of Nazi Germany, in the Pioneer youth movements of the former Soviet Union and its satellite states, in youth Pioneer programmes in China and Vietnam, as well as in the independence struggles of many African countries.

Today, in countries such as Australia, Canada, the United Kingdom and the United States, young people occupy an ambiguous position. On the one hand, they are viewed as potentially threatening (of violence, of insubordination and of change); on the other hand they are seen as holding rich potential for the future. The term *adolescence,* so beloved of psychologists and public health specialists, itself captures many of these tensions. In North America, and particularly in the United States, the term is often used normatively to highlight a stage of life young people pass through en route to a supposedly stable and responsible adulthood. In the United Kingdom and Australia, however, the term is often eschewed because of its tendency to homogenize and pathologize all young people and because of its strongly negative connotations. More neutral terms such as *youth* and *young people* tend to be preferred, the latter because of the stress it places on personhood and rights. Ultimately, however, all definitions of adolescence and youth are socially constructed – in line with particular taken-for-granted assumptions or ideologies, which are themselves deeply rooted in history. We should be careful therefore in their use, lest we come to take as 'fact' that which is culturally, ideologically and socially determined.

But where do such images and ideas come from, and what purpose do they serve? A persuasive account was offered by the Canadian academic and psychotherapist Elisabeth Young-Bruehl (2009), whose work highlights three types of 'prejudicial image' underpinning negative responses to children. The first of these portrays children as intrinsically evil, the bearers of original sin. According to Young-Bruehl, such a view is often held by 'obsessional' people who see children as pollutants, monopolizing and contaminating society. G. Stanley Hall perhaps shared this sentiment in his characterization of preadolescent children as 'savages' and in his advocacy of charismatic leadership to manipulate their 'herd instincts'. A second image of childhood and youth, often adhered to by those displaying 'narcissism', considers children a threat. Not only do young people rebel against their parents and elders, but they also reject tradition and must therefore be brought into line. Within this framing, children are viewed as little more than their parents' or the community's possessions, ready to be shaped to what the wider society requires. A third image, said to be common amongst those of a 'hysterical' type, promotes an understanding of children as the 'repositories of sexual energy, youthful vigor, lasciviousness, [and] seductiveness' (Young-Bruehl 2009, p. 261). Young people therefore need to be controlled and submitted to various forms of sexual restriction. As Greslé-Favier (2013) perceptively has argued, such a perspective 'coexists with a negation of these images through the construction of children as innocent, asexual, clean and non-polluting'.[1]

In a recent paper, Rijk van Dijk, Mirjam de Bruijn, Carlos Cordoso and Inge Butter (2011) examined a number of different ideologies of youth as revealed in the health and development literatures. They began by noting once more the socially constructed nature of youth; its close connections to notions of risk; and the linking of young people to the causes and solutions to social, economic and political problems. Increasingly, the period of life that counts as youth is becoming extended. This favours an understanding of youth as an identity project of 'becoming somebody', pursued by navigating certain spaces: 'the bar, the disco, the funeral, the school, the church, the state, the house and so forth' (*ibid.*, p. 6). The concept of 'youthscapes' may prove useful in understanding the ambiguous locations young people occupy between local contexts, national ideologies and global markets (*ibid.*, p. 6; but see also Maira and Soep 2004), and describes the social spaces in which being young and living through new experiences provide opportunity for self-understanding and identity formation.

Young people also constitute a powerful ideological force in and of themselves. Their role in nation-building and postcolonial struggle has been well documented (Abbink and van Kesell 2005), but young people are not infrequently viewed as threats to the prevailing social order and the harbingers of unpredictable forms of social change (Hall and Jefferson 1993). Hence there is a need for leadership and what may be seen as 'adult-ist' forms of control. Crucially, young people are not the passive victims of the constraint that is imposed on them. Instead, through contestation and resistance, they engage with, modify, mutate and transform the material and symbolic resources at their disposal, creating new social practices and meanings as the result of this. But what are the implications of such a position for young people's health and for health promotion?

In this volume, Grace Spencer engages with these and related issues. Taking as her starting point young people's own beliefs and practices, and questioning the orthodoxy that suggests that young people lack power to effect health-promoting change, this book offers a positive perspective on what needs to be done. Following a detailed interrogation of what power may actually mean in young people's lives, the book focuses on what young people actually understand is meant by 'health'. The importance of happiness comes out centrally in the accounts informants provide, pointing to the salience of emotional well-being for emic as well as in more distanced (Graham 2008) appreciations of the social determinants of health. Young people describe frequently being talked down to by others and being misunderstood, with major implications for health promotion, particularly if we are to move beyond the impositional, top-down approaches that are so often used. *Empowerment, Health Promotion and Young People* points to innovative ways of working with young people, in which 'partnership' and 'participation' move beyond rhetoric to become grounded in young people's diverse experiences, circumstances and lives.

Peter Aggleton
UNSW Strategic Professor in Education and Health
The University of New South Wales, Sydney, Australia
May 2013

References

Abbink, J. and van Kesell, I. (2005). (eds.) *Vanguards and Vandals: Youth politics and conflict in Africa*. Leiden, the Netherlands: Brill.

Addams, J. (1909). *The Spirit of Youth and the City Streets*. New York, NY: Macmillan.

Ariès, P. (1962). Centuries of Childhood. New York, NY: Vintage Books.

Curtis, C. (2013). Be Part of the Next Four Years. Whitehouse Blog. [Online]. Available at: http://www.whitehouse.gov/blog/2013/01/21/be-part-next-four-years [Last accessed May 2013].

Graham, C. (2008). 'Happiness And Health: Lessons – And Questions – For Public Policy'. *Health Affairs*, 27, (1), 72–87.

Greslé-Favier, C. (2013). 'Adult discrimination against children: the case of abstinence-only education in 21st century USA'. *Sex Education*. http://dx.doi.org/10.1080/14681811.2013.813387.

Hall, G.S. (1904). *Adolescence – Its Psychology and Its Relations to Physiology, Anthropology, Sociology, Sex, Crime, and Religion*. (vols. I and II). New York, NY: Appleton.

Hall, S. and Jefferson, T. (eds.) (1993). *Resistance through Rituals: Youth Subcultures in Postwar Britain*. London, UK: Routledge, Chapman and Hall.

Karrier, C.J. (1986). *The Individual, Society, and Education: A History of American Educational Ideas*. Urbana: University of Illinois Press.

Maira, S. and Soep, W. (eds.) (2004). *Youthscapes: The Popular, the National, the Global*. Philadelphia: University of Pennsylvania Press.

van Dijk, R., de Bruijn, M., Cordoso, C. and Butter, I. (2011). 'Introduction: Ideologies of Youth'. *Africa Development*, 36, (3–4), 1–17.

Young-Bruehl, E. (2009). Childism: prejudice against children. *Contemporary Psychoanalysis*, 45, (2), 251–265.

Preface

A number of experiences provide the impetus for a book on empowerment, health promotion and young people. Specifically, this book is informed by many of the insights gleaned from more than 15 years of grappling with some of the theoretical complexities (and contradictions) surrounding current uses of empowerment within the field of health promotion. In particular, the book draws on key findings and knowledge developed from my own doctoral work that sought to better understand the concept of empowerment as it relates to young people and their health (Spencer 2011). These insights and understandings offer a more critical approach to the exploration of empowerment than hitherto articulated in the existing literature, thus helping to enhance both the theorization of empowerment and also its more meaningful use in health promotion practice with young people.

My own interest in the concept of empowerment commenced during my undergraduate studies in nursing. At that time, I was introduced to some of the complexities of promoting health, including some of the extensively documented structural and contextual features that generate and sustain health-related inequalities and inequities (Townsend and Davidson 1982, Whitehead 1988, Dahlgren and Whitehead 1991, Wilkinson 1996, Acheson 1998). I was particularly drawn to critical social theory and inspired by the works of Antonio Gramsci (1971), Paulo Freire (1970, 1996), Steven Lukes (1974, 2005) and Michel Foucault (1980, 1990), amongst others. As an undergraduate student, I saw great merit in analysing these theorists in line with current debates on health promotion and, more specifically, the concept of empowerment – which at that time was gaining increasing popularity following a number of international reports on health promotion (World Health Organization [WHO] 1977, 1986).

As part of my undergraduate studies I undertook a critical analysis of the concept of empowerment. Drawing on theorizations of power, in this early work I began to draw out and interrogate some of the thorny theoretical tensions and unquestioned assumptions surrounding concepts of empowerment. More specifically, this work addressed the potential significance of the social category of *age*; which at that time, I felt this had received little attention as a key structuring determinant of health and as an important unit of social analysis, alongside other more commonly theorized and investigated dimensions, such as those linked to social class, gender and ethnicity.

Building on this conceptual background, during postgraduate research I began (albeit rather tentatively) to empirically investigate the 'meaning' of empowerment in relation to young people's health and their health-related practices. In this work, I examined young people's perceptions of health, risk and UK government priority areas such as smoking, drinking and healthy eating (Department of Health [DH] 2004a). Taking this work further, subsequent postgraduate research similarly focused on young people's perspectives on health-related risks, examining too some of the relative strengths and limitations of various research methods in accessing young people's views on concepts of health and health-related risk.

Coupled with these theoretical interests, when I was working as a nurse, I often saw how public health priority areas, such as smoking, alcohol use, healthy eating, physical activity and sexual health, appeared somewhat detached from the everyday concerns and experiences of young people (Wills *et al.* 2008, Woodgate and Leach 2010). This was illustrated on a number of occasions whilst delivering health education in schools in England. The questions asked by young people, for example, 'Is it ok to be homophobic?', 'What causes spots?', and 'Is it ok to fight with someone?' often represented concerns that reached beyond official health prescriptions.

Such questions highlighted how young people differ considerably in their perspectives, practices and experiences. Not all young people are the same; when it comes to health orientations, there exist systematic differences, for example, between the experiences of young women and young men; between young people of differing sexualities; and between young people from different social class backgrounds (Aggleton and Campbell 2000, Shoveller *et al.* 2004). Understanding young people's own perspectives and experiences of health is thus paramount if future health promotion efforts are to be consistent with how young people themselves perceive their health. Without this insight, not only does health promotion run the risk of seeming irrelevant to young people but arguably undermines many of the original underpinning principles of empowerment that stress the importance of identifying people's own concerns (Laverack 2009).

Of particular relevance to my interest in empowerment and young people's health was the time spent working on a number of empowerment-based projects in various international settings including Tanzania, Brazil and South Africa. Working with community members on projects underpinned and informed by concepts of empowerment often revealed some of the complexities of translating theoretical ideals into practice. Within these diverse contexts, concepts of empowerment were, and continue to be, positively advocated as a positive, proactive and 'bottom-up' strategy to health promotion. However, little is known about the mechanisms through which empowerment might lead to (positive) health, or indeed the potential and diverse ways in which dominant power relations come to shape and define the possibilities for, and limitations of, empowerment within any given context.

Whilst more individualized notions of the concept of empowerment have been adopted within much recent UK health promotion practice, often based on the development of young people's self-esteem and confidence (see DH 2004a, 2010a), more collective forms of the concept stem from the work of the Brazilian educationalist Paulo Freire and his discussion of *conscientização* or critical consciousness raising (Freire 1996). To observe some of these conceptual differences, in 2006 I made the decision to volunteer as a nurse on an empowerment-based community development project in a large *favela* in Rio de Janeiro. During this time, it became quickly apparent how young people's experiences of health and empowerment were inextricably bound with the effects of poverty, mediated through the activity of drug trafficking. In this context, the intricate workings of power came to the fore as young people's daily activities appeared to be shaped not by more individualized processes of self-esteem and confidence but through the various collective strategies they developed to negotiate the very real dangers presented by the daily operation of drug trafficking (cf. Zaluar 2001, Zdun 2008).

Building on these experiences in Brazil, I subsequently worked as a nurse volunteer in South Africa on an empowerment-based HIV project with young people. In this context, the interplay of poverty *and* gender were particularly pronounced, yet these projects, like many others, remained committed to promoting (individualized) aspects of young people's self-esteem and confidence as evidence of their 'empowerment' (see Morton and Montgomery 2011). Whilst not downplaying the very real importance of supporting young people in feeling positive about who they are and what they do, this sustained focus on concepts linked to self-esteem often fails to fully engage with the structural and contextual factors that shape the health and everyday lives of young people (Aggleton and Campbell 2000, Goldenberg *et al.* 2008, Shoveller *et al.* 2004, 2010).

Participating in such projects not only fuelled my enthusiasm for this area of work but also generated considerable frustration as different notions of empowerment seemed to be used rather inconsistently and with very limited account of the ways in which dominant relations of power may shape the possibilities for, and limitations of, empowerment. The absence of an understanding of power seemed to oversimplify the relationship between empowerment and health, with the overriding assumption that empowerment unproblematically translates into positive health outcomes.

Observing the diversity of young people's experiences in varying international settings not only signalled to me the growing disjunction between 'official' and 'lay' perspectives on health (see for example, Lupton 2005, Blaxter 2010) but also seemed to reflect a broader tendency to homogenize and pathologize young people (Kelly 2006). The disjunction between protectionist and participatory discourses[1] in much existing literature on young people's health, along with the marginalization of young people's own perspectives, provided the rationale for exploring and problematizing this aspect of health promotion as part of my doctoral work. My doctoral dissertation, which this book draws from, focused closely on the concept of empowerment as it relates to young people's health (Spencer 2011). Specifically, the goal of the investigation was to better understand what might be the possibilities for, and limitations of, empowerment amongst young people through a close-focused analysis of the related concept of *power*.

These experiences, and many others, provide the context and inspiration for this book. Drawing together key debates and thinking, this book aims to examine more critically the concept of empowerment and consider its relationship to young people's health and crucially, from a perspective of power. An investigation of this kind offers the possibility for new theoretical insight in this field, as well as the development of opportunities for future (more theoretically informed) approaches to health promotion based on concepts of empowerment.

Acknowledgements

There are many people I would like to thank for their support, inspiration and critical commentaries on the development of this work. In particular, this work draws on my doctoral dissertation undertaken at the Thomas Coram Research Unit, Institute of Education, University of London and funded by a 1+3 studentship award from the Economic and Social Research Council (ESRC). I am enormously grateful to my supervisors – Peter Aggleton and Claire Maxwell. Their timely commitment and critical comments served to deepen both my thinking and my enthusiasm for this work. Thanks must also go to Jean Shoveller and her team at School of Population and Public Health, University of British Columbia, Canada. The support and kindness offered has been of inestimable value to the successful completion of this book. Huge thanks goes to Marion Doull and Kate Greany for proofreading and providing detailed comments on earlier versions of the book. This work would have not been possible without the enthusiastic contributions and commitment of all the young people involved in the study. I am especially grateful to all the school staff and other professionals who took time to be involved in discussions and who were instrumental in ensuring the overall success of the study. A special thanks goes to my parents, who have always supported me unconditionally, and to my husband Andrew, who endured constant disruptions to our wedding plans during the final stages of the doctorate and then again, whilst drafting final versions of this book. Finally, I would like to acknowledge Sage Publishing Limited and the Emerald Publishing Group for granting permissions to reproduce and reprint previously published versions of this work.

Part I

Empowerment, health promotion and young people

1 Introduction

Empowerment is widely considered to be one of the primary goals of health promotion (World Health Organization [WHO] 1986, Tones 1998a and b, 2001, Tones and Tilford 2001, Wallerstein 2002, 2006, Laverack 2004, 2007, 2009, Wiggins 2011). Concepts of empowerment now feature strongly in public health discourses on young people's health (Department of Health [DH] 2010b, Australian Institute of Health and Welfare [AIHW] 2011, WHO 2011b), amidst increasing concerns about young people's engagement in 'risky' health-related practices such as smoking, drinking alcohol, unhealthy eating and sexual activity. Globally, the health of young people has attracted much attention in recent years. The WHO (2011b), for example, stresses the importance of promoting positive health practices and reducing health risks during adolescence – highlighting too, the right to health for all young people, as enshrined within the United Nations Convention on the Rights of the Child (UNCRC) (United Nations [UN] Assembly 1989).

This recent growing concern about young people's health has triggered a wealth of initiatives that seek to 'empower' young people to take control of (and responsibility for) their own health (see for example, Helve and Wallace 2001, Berman 2003, Altman and Feighery 2004, Wight and Dixon 2004, Jennings *et al.* 2006, Berg, Coman and Schensul 2009, Pearrow and Pollock 2009, Mohajer and Earnest 2009, 2010). Despite (or perhaps because of) its popularity, the concept of empowerment remains undertheorized and its relationship to young people's health less well understood. This book on empowerment, health promotion and young people therefore aims to better understand the relationship between empowerment and young people's health. Specifically, the book addresses some of the (unquestioned) assumptions and contradictions surrounding current uses of empowerment and, by doing so, seeks to advance the conceptualization of empowerment and enhance its more meaningful use in health promotion with young people. Toward these goals, a new conceptual framework for understanding the concept of empowerment as it relates to young people's health is proposed (see Chapter Eight). Drawing together key contributions from the literature to date and findings from an empirical enquiry on young people's health, this new framework helps to better unpack the relationship between empowerment and health – offering some new and critical insights into the field of young people's health and health promotion more broadly.

Before detailing some of the book's main arguments, it is important to highlight how the approach taken in this book may differ from some of the existing contributions in the field. First, this book adopts a more critical approach to understanding the concept of empowerment than hitherto articulated in the health promotion literature; specifically the book troubles the widely held assumption that processes of empowerment unproblematically translate into positive health outcomes. Taking different perspectives of *power* as its starting point, the book's theoretical depth and criticality provide a more theoretically informed and nuanced analysis of the conceptualization of empowerment. By doing so, the book aims to scrutinize more thoroughly some of the rarely addressed thorny theoretical tensions and operational challenges surrounding current uses of the term in the field of health promotion and specifically, in relation to young people and their health.

Second, unlike much of the literature on young people's health, this book positions young people's frames of reference as being central to understanding the concept of empowerment and its relationship to, and relevance for, young people's health. Consequently, the focus here is on *health* as defined by young people themselves – in contrast to adopting a more predefined approach led by health priority areas, such as smoking, drinking alcohol, drug use, physical activity, healthy eating and so forth. By foregrounding young people's own frames of reference when discussing health, some of the existing (more negative) ways of understanding young people's health are challenged – revealing too how these alternative conceptions of health are intricately linked to, and underpinned by, notions of power.

The main focus of this introductory chapter is to set out some of the book's key arguments, which are further interrogated in subsequent chapters. In particular, this first chapter highlights the increasing popularity of the concept of empowerment in the broad field of health promotion and, more specifically, its use in relation to young people's health. The chapter charts some of the recent political and public concern about young people's health and specifically, their engagement with 'risky' health-related behaviours. Four key arguments are outlined here.

First, as suggested, I argue that despite its popularity, the concept of empowerment has been poorly conceptualized in much of the literature, and its relationship to young people's health is currently not well understood. In particular, notions of empowerment are frequently presented as 'solutions' to the 'problem' of young people's health, often without critical attention to the concept's theoretical underpinnings or indeed to the related concepts of *power*.

Second, the failure to adequately conceptualize empowerment has resulted in many inconsistencies in the way the concept has been used both within policy and research with young people. These inconsistencies in use not only lead to the assumption that empowerment unproblematically translates into positive health outcomes, but also point to an emerging disjunction between the participatory and protectionist discourses that guide much health promotion practice with young people.

Third, I argue that by emphasizing risks to young people's health, much recent health-related policy has taken a largely predefined and protectionist risk-reduction approach. Not only does this predefined approach appear to be antithetical to the concept of empowerment (which focuses on identifying people's own concerns and priorities for health; see Labonte 1989, 1994, Laverack 2004, 2009), but I further argue that dominant health discourses based on reducing young people's engagement with risky health practices downplays crucial evidence highlighting some of the different meanings and understandings young people attach to their health and health-related practices (Brooks and Magnusson 2007, Spencer 2008, Wills *et al.* 2008). The intention here is not to simply 'explain away' the risks associated with particular health behaviours but to better understand these practices within the context of young people's everyday lives and, crucially, the implications they may hold for furthering the understanding of empowerment.

Fourth and finally, by examining young people's 'alternative' perspectives on health (including the factors young people themselves see as promoting or constraining their health) the purported health-enhancing outcomes of empowerment may be challenged. Young people's potentially alternative ways of seeing and experiencing health, however, open possibilities for some new and differing understandings of empowerment – as later chapters reveal. The final part of this introductory chapter outlines the overall structure to the book and how these identified issues will be subsequently addressed.

Empowerment, health promotion and young people

Globally, young people's health is an increasing priority area for health practitioners, policymakers and researchers. Concern about young people's health and, in particular, the health-related risks associated with smoking, drinking, unhealthy eating, drug use, and sexual activity is frequently reported in popular media and features strongly in international literatures and policy discourses on young people's health (see for example United Nations Children's Fund 2007, DH 2010b, AIHW 2011, WHO 2011b).

In the UK context, for example, issues such as teenage pregnancy, binge-drinking and obesity have attracted many negative commentaries in recent years – prompting what has been described as a wider 'moral panic' about young people and varying aspects of their health and well-being (Campos *et al.* 2006, Arai 2009, Morrow and Mayall 2009, Macvarish 2010, Monaghan and Malson 2013). A similar outlook on young people's health exists in Canada, where, for example, rates of sexually transmitted infections and alcohol misuse continue to escalate, particularly amongst socially disadvantaged population subgroups of young people (Smith, Martin and the McCreary Centre Society 2010). Likewise, in Australia, young people's health and specifically their engagement in risky health practices is a central focus in recent public health discourses:

> 'Too many young people are overweight or obese, not meeting physical activity or fruit and vegetable guidelines, are drinking at risky or high-risk levels for short-term or long-term harm, are victims of alcohol- or drug-related violence or are homeless' (AIHW 2011, p vii).

Concepts of empowerment are frequently presented as a solution to the 'problem' of young people's health (Wight and Dixon 2004, Mohajer and Earnest 2009, 2010, Pearrow and Pollock 2009, DH 2010b, Morton and Montgomery 2011), with the assumption being made that empowerment translates unproblematically into reduced health risks and more positive health outcomes. The National Strategy for Young Australians (Australian Government 2010), for example, sets out the Australian Government's vision for promoting young people's health through 'empowering young people to build their own lives . . . and to take part and be active in their communities' (p. 3). This document further outlines the Australian Government's plans to minimize health risks through the use of

> social marketing techniques to equip young people with information to help them avoid risks and harm associated with a range of behaviours including smoking, unsafe sex, binge-drinking and illicit drug use, and to emphasize harms associated with ecstasy, cannabis and ice.[1] (p. 14)

Likewise in the UK, the previous Labour government's[2] health policy *Choosing Health: Making Healthy Choices Easier* (DH 2004a) gave specific attention to young people and sought to 'strengthen measures to protect children and young people and help them understand and manage risk and develop responsible patterns of behaviour' (DH 2004a, p. 41). The Department of Health, drawing in many ways on the participatory principles of the UNCRC (UN Assembly 1989), argued that promoting young people's health would be achieved through building 'a culture of participation where children and young people are involved in the range of issues and decisions that affect them' (DH 2004a, p. 48).

The successive and more recently formed coalition government[3] in the UK further stresses a 'radical approach' to public health based on the empowerment of communities (DH 2010b, p. 2). Young people attract specific attention as being the 'biggest lifestyle risk-takers' and the identified priority is the need to strengthen their self-esteem, confidence and resilience to 'empower them to make healthy choices' (DH 2010b, p. 6).

By stressing the risks to young people's health, not only do these policy discourses fuel widespread (negative) concern about young people and their health (Kelly 2000, 2003, 2006, Messias *et al.* 2008, Austen 2009), and specifically their risky health behaviours, but they also appear to advocate for a notion of empowerment that seems somewhat inconsistent with many of its original theoretical underpinnings. As further detailed in Chapter Two, many of these original interpretations of empowerment stress the importance of a 'bottom-up' strategy based on people's own concerns (Labonte 1989, 1994) and place particular emphasis on notions of autonomy, collectivism and resistance (Barker 1999, Labonte 1993, Wallerstein 2002, Laverack 2004, 2009, Eyben and Napier-Moore 2009, Wiggins 2011).

Consequently, whilst advocating for young people's empowerment, this policy emphasis (and related areas of health promotion practice) seems to adopt a more predefined risk-reduction approach that appears antithetical to the concept of empowerment itself in its failure to try and understand and take seriously young people's own perspectives on health. This (more negative) risk-based approach further downplays possibilities for a more positive conceptualization of young people and their health (Ingham 2006) – an understanding of which may be paramount to the possibilities for empowerment amongst young people.

The widespread global attention on young people's health and health-risks has led to a proliferation of research that has sought to identify young people's perspectives on their health (see for example Armstrong, Hill and Secker 2000, Ioannou 2003, 2009, van Exel, de Graaf and Brouwer 2006, Woodgate and Leach 2010, Nelson, MacDonald and Abbott 2012). This body of research, however, has typically been framed according to official priority areas such as sexual health (see Skidmore and Hayter 2000, Hyde *et al.* 2005, Stanley 2005), alcohol (see Bogren 2006, Järvinen and Gundelach 2007, Tutenges and Rod 2009, Järvinen 2012), smoking (see Denscombe 2001a and b, Turner and Gordon 2004, Haines, Poland and Johnson 2009), drug use (see Hunt, Evans and Kares 2007, Pilkington 2007), mental health (see Armstrong, Hill and Secker 2000, Johansson, Brunnberg and Eriksson 2007), physical activity (see Brooks and Magnusson 2007, Gosling, Stanistreet and Swami 2008, Nelson, MacDonald and Abbott 2012) and healthy eating and obesity (see Dixey *et al.* 2001, Bauer, Yang and Austin 2004, Ioannou 2009, Ridder *et al.* 2010, Rees *et al.* 2011).

Whilst providing important insights into young people's thoughts on various health topics, rarely has this strand of research sought to identify young people's own understandings of health more broadly or the potentially different areas young people identify as pertinent to their health (exceptions include Aggleton *et al.* 1996, 1998, Spencer 2008, 2013a and b). Starting from young people's own perspectives on health is a necessary step to ensure future health promotion efforts are consistent with how young people themselves perceive and experience health (Aggleton and Campbell 2000). Without this insight, not only does health promotion run the risk of seeming irrelevant to young people but again seems to undermine the more bottom-up principles of empowerment that stress the importance of identifying and working from people's own (health-related) concerns (Labonte 1989, 1994, Laverack 2009).

The relative lack of attention given to young people's own frames of reference in terms of health is particularly pertinent given the now growing body of evidence that suggests current public health priority areas may not resonate with young people's own understandings of health and their health-related concerns (Percy-Smith 2006, 2007, Brooks and Magnusson 2007, Sixsmith *et al.* 2007, Spencer 2008, Wills *et al.* 2008, Woodgate and Leach 2010). In particular, this related area of research highlights the relevance of some of the more socially contingent meanings young people attach to health and their health-related practices (see France 2000, Mitchell *et al.* 2001, Tulloch and Lupton 2003, Shoveller *et al.* 2004, 2010, Ingham 2006, Marston, King and Ingham 2006, Austen 2009, Stead *et al.* 2011, Nelson, MacDonald and Abbott 2012). Several studies now point to evidence of the positive and pleasurable aspects of taking up health-related practices defined as 'risky' by official health discourses (Lupton and Tulloch 2002, Stanley 2005, Gilbert 2007, Lindsay 2009, Tutenges and Rod 2009, Harrison *et al.* 2011, Järvinen 2012).

Arguably, evidence of this kind may in fact point to young people's increasing autonomy (Katainen 2006), resistance (Raby 2010) and 'empowerment' (Denscombe 2001a) as they actively *choose* to engage in practices identified as 'risky' by official health discourse, irrespective (and often in full knowledge) of the health risks presented (Denscombe 2001a, Baillie *et al.* 2005, Katainen 2006). Young people's resistance to official forms of health promotion not only questions the widespread assumption that empowerment will result in positive health outcomes (as defined by dominant public health discourses) but further exemplifies how current uses of the term *empowerment* have become increasingly removed from many of the concept's original theoretical underpinnings.

Outline of the book

The emergent contradictions and underlying assumptions in policy and health promotion literature set out here highlight a need to better address the theoretical complexity surrounding concepts of empowerment as they relate to young people's health. The chapters that follow seek to address these tensions more fully and crucially and better explain the relationship between empowerment and young people's health.

The book is in two main parts. Part One provides the theoretical framework and details some of the key theoretical contributions made to the existing literature on empowerment. In particular, Part One of the book examines differing conceptions of power and empowerment and how these concepts have been variously defined and used in relation to young people's health and health promotion practice. Part Two draws from this theoretical base and details an empirical investigation on power, empowerment and young people's health. The main aim of this empirical investigation was to examine the possibilities for, and limitations of, empowerment amongst young people (Spencer 2011). Here, a new conceptual framework for understanding empowerment as it relates to young people's health is proposed (see also Spencer 2013a).

This first chapter has introduced Part One of the book and some of the emerging tensions arising from existing uses of concepts of empowerment in health promotion policy and practice. Chapter Two then explores these tensions more fully by examining the diverse meanings and uses of empowerment in the literature. Specifically, Chapter Two argues that underpinning concepts of empowerment are the related concepts of *power* – an understanding of which may point to differing possibilities for, and limitations of, empowerment amongst young people.

Chapter Three takes up the discussion on power in several ways. A number of differing perspectives on power are given, and their implications for understanding the related concept of empowerment are considered. In particular, Steven Lukes's (1974, 2005) tripartite of power is examined to highlight its potential to offer a more nuanced and critical insight into the concept of empowerment. Lukes's perspective of power is especially appropriate in this regard because it provides a framework that integrates the multiple ways power has been conceptualized and operates at individual, structural and ideological levels. This framework brings to the fore some of the theoretical tensions within the concept of empowerment from varying interpretations of power and further forms a key part of the investigation outlined in Part Two of the book. Chapter Three then concludes with a close-focused examination of the possibilities for, and limitations of, empowerment amongst young people as given in the existing literature from the aforementioned tripartite perspective of power (*power to, power over, power through*).

Chapter Four introduces Part Two of the book by describing the overall methodological approach to an empirical enquiry that sought to more thoroughly examine and operationalize the theoretical tensions outlined in Part One. Key methodological concerns and the potential complexities of conducting research with young people are also considered. The chapter provides important details about the study design and methods employed to investigate the concept of empowerment as it relates to young people's health.

Chapters Five, Six and Seven present some of the key findings from the empirical enquiry (see also Spencer 2011, 2013a, b and c). Specifically, Chapter Five analyses young people's understandings of *health*, including their accounts of feeling well. As the analysis that follows illuminates, these accounts challenge existing (individualized) understandings of empowerment in the health promotion literature. Chapter Six continues with a close-focused analysis of young people's perspectives on 'not feeling well', including the specific issues and factors young people themselves identify as negatively affecting their health. Chapter Seven concludes the focus on empirical data by examining young people's priorities for health promotion and how these suggestions might help inform future health promotion efforts *with* young people to bring about social change in line with their own perspectives on health.

Chapter Eight draws together the empirical findings and, informed by Lukes's (1974, 2005) tripartite model of power, proposes a new conceptual framework for understanding the concept of empowerment as it relates to young people's health. This new framework helps better explain some of the thorny theoretical tensions within existing conceptualizations of empowerment and, importantly, the relationship between empowerment and young people's health. Here, six new forms of empowerment are developed (*impositional, dispositional, concessional, oppositional, normative and transformative*) based on differing perspectives of health (*dominant* and *alternative*) and underpinned by differing conceptions of power (*power to, power over, power through*).

Finally, the book's concluding chapter underscores the book's contribution to existing debates on empowerment, health promotion and young people more broadly. This includes a critical reflection on some of the challenges involved in the investigation of young people's health – offering some possibilities for future enquiry in this field. Implications for further theorizations of empowerment and health promotion practice and policy are also identified. This includes a discussion of the implications the presenting framework may hold for young people's health, along with a broader consideration of health promotion with other groups, such as adults, younger children and minority groups from differing social and cultural backgrounds and contexts.

2 The diverse meanings of empowerment

This chapter explores the concept of empowerment and its different meanings and uses in the literature. Building on the arguments in the book's introduction, the first part of this chapter charts the increasing popularity and use of empowerment across a range of literatures and disciplines and, specifically, within the field of health promotion. Particular attention is given to the use of empowerment in relation to young people's health and the ways in which the concept has been drawn upon in much recent public health policy and health promotion practice to encourage young people to adopt 'expert' defined 'healthy' behaviours. Here, I argue that many current uses of empowerment often lack grounding in theoretically informed and consistent definitions. Examining these inconsistencies in use brings to the fore a number of theoretical tensions and contradictions when considering the concept's relationship to young people's health and health promotion policy and practice more broadly.

The next section of this chapter then offers a critical review of the diverse ways in which empowerment has been conceptualized in the field of health promotion. My aim here is to tease out some of the important conceptual features of empowerment, which are then further interrogated in relation to young people's experiences of health in Part Two of the book. Conceptual distinctions are made between empowerment as a process and/or as an outcome and between *individual* or psychological empowerment and *community* or collective forms of empowerment. The chapter reveals how much of the existing literature on young people's health continues to advocate the concept of empowerment without clear conceptualization of the word itself and critically, its root word – *power* (the focus of the following chapter).

Empowerment – Its different meanings and uses

Definitions of empowerment vary considerably across a range of literatures. The concept of empowerment now features strongly as a popular concern for a number of disciplines and practices, including social work (see Pease 2002, Thompson 2002, 2007, Gaiswinkler and Roessler 2009), nursing (see Skelton 1994, Gilbert 1995, Anderson 1996, Rodwell 1996, Chang, Liu and Yen 2008, Ning *et al.* 2009), organization and management studies (see Lee and Koh 2001, Lincoln *et al.* 2002, Gill *et al.* 2010), feminism and feminist practice (see Karl 1995, Mosedale 2005, Peterson 2010, Sardenberg 2010), disability studies (see Barnes and Mercer 1995, Yeoh 2009), critical race studies (see Stovall 2006, Briggs 2010), childhood studies (see Cook 2007, Qvortrup, Corsaro and Honig 2009) and international development literatures (see United Nations Population Fund 2006, Gibson and Woolcock 2008, Eyben and Napier-Moore 2009, Kuttab, 2010).

Within the field of management studies, for example, the concept of empowerment is presented as being both a process and an outcome and, according to these perspectives, is evident in examples of increases in employee work motivation, productivity, job performance and satisfaction (Lee and Koh, 2001, Lincoln *et al.* 2002). Through the process of empowerment, employees develop an increasing sense of control (and thus, responsibility for work-related tasks and decision-making). Critiques of these interpretations of empowerment, however, have pointed to the ways in which these forms of decision-making remain largely set within (and constrained by) hierarchical management structures and organizational goals (Lee and Koh 2001). Such usages of empowerment have therefore been criticized for creating a false rhetoric of 'empowerment' that ultimately supports employee exploitation for capitalist gain (see Kuokkanen and Katajisto 2003).

In a contrasting area of literature, definitions of empowerment drawn from varying strands of feminism note the centrality of gender relations and women's agency – often highlighting the importance of developing women's *power within* to bring about social change. In an early definition of women's empowerment as 'adding to women's power', Griffen (1987, p. 117) emphasized women's participation within decision-making processes. Other more recent contributions to these feminist perspectives have drawn attention to examples of so-called 'girl power' and 'ladette' cultures as evidence of young girls' (sexual) agency and empowerment (see for example Currie, Kelly and Pomerantz 2006, 2011, Jackson 2006, Petersen 2010, Doull and Sethna 2011). This body of literature points to evidence of some women and girls who appear to express a new 'emancipated femininity' (Lazar 2011) through displaying their independence, autonomy and 'empowerment' (Duits and van Zoonen 2006, Currie, Kelly and Pomerantz 2011, Doull and Sethna 2011, Harvey and Gill 2011). Whilst such evidence of 'girl power' has proliferated in recent times, others have rejected these expressions of empowerment as an indicator of women's (increasing) power (see for example Gill 2007a and b, 2008, 2009), and instead highlight how these young women's expressions of power ultimately remain set within dominant gendered power relations (see for example, Allen 2003a and b, Gill 2007a and b, 2008, 2009).

The nursing literature has also given significant attention to the concept of empowerment (Gibson 1991, Skelton 1994, Gilbert 1995, Anderson 1996, Rodwell 1996, Ryles 1999, Bradbury-Jones, Sambrook and Irvine

2008, Chang, Liu and Yen 2008). This body of literature and area of practice typically advocates the notion of empowerment as a means through which nurses themselves can advance their occupational position for the purported benefit of patients' health and well-being. This understanding of empowerment is widely echoed in recent UK health policy that places significant emphasis on empowering frontline staff, such as doctors and nurses, in order to enhance the quality and delivery of patient care (Department of Health [DH] 2010a). However, rarely do such discussions offer examples of how empowerment may be achieved in practice or indeed, acknowledge the related issues of power that place nurses themselves in a relatively powerless position within the health care system (Kendall 1998, Latter 1998). This relatively powerless position may well set limits to any potential for both patient and nurses' empowerment (Salvage 1992). These more 'top-down' and often highly individualistic approaches to empowerment have thus been widely criticized for simply reflecting a series of occupational strategies that ultimately seek to advance the professionalization of nursing, thereby supporting nurses', rather than patients', interests (Porter 1992, Salvage 1992, Manojlovich 2007), a criticism echoed elsewhere in the literature in relation to social work (Pease 2002) and education practice (Gillman 1996).

Historically, the concept of empowerment has been widely considered to be one of the primary goals of health promotion and, more recently, within the 'new public health' (Rappaport 1984, World Health Organization [WHO] 1986, Ashton and Seymour 1988, Labonte 1989, 1994, Farrant 1991, Zimmerman 1995, Tones 1998a, 2001, Tones and Tilford 2001, Wallerstein 2002, 2006, Laverack 2007, 2009). The concept features strongly in recent public health discourses, and empowerment now appears as a key element of much international health promotion practice, policy and research (Kendall 1998, Tones 1998a and b, Laverack and Wallerstein 2001, Tones and Tilford 2001, Wallerstein 2002, 2006, Laverack 2004, 2007, Tengland 2007, 2008, Braunack-Mayer and Louise 2008, Pearrow and Pollack 2009, DH 2010b, Laverack and Whipple 2010, Wiggins 2011).

Evidence of the concept's increasing popularity in the broad field of health promotion can be seen in the extension of a number of empowerment-based initiatives targeting a diverse range of different population subgroups in varying country contexts. Examples of such include children and young people living in contexts of poverty (Karmaliani *et al.* 2009, Ssewamala *et al.* 2012), the elderly (Minkler 1985, Hage and Lorensen 2005), individuals with long-term health conditions and disabilities (Chang, Li and Lu 2004, Jingree and Finlay 2012), female sex workers (see Blanchard *et al.* 2013, Weine *et al.* 2013) and women at risk of HIV infection (Romero *et al.* 2006), men who have sex with men (Crossley 2001a, Fields *et al.* 2012) and with individuals living in contexts of family or domestic violence (Kelly *et al.* 2007, Krishnan *et al.* 2012).

The increasing popularity of empowerment in the field of health promotion was most notably endorsed (and evidenced) by various WHO statements, including the Alma Ata Declaration (WHO 1977), Ottawa Charter (WHO 1986) and the more recent Bangkok Charter (WHO 2005). The Ottawa Charter, for example, explicitly identified community action and empowerment as central components of health promotion practice and a means through which communities can take ownership and control over their own lives (WHO 1986). Drawing particular attention to the interrelationship between health and the socioeconomic environment, much of the mainstream health promotion literature presents and advocates empowerment as a positive and proactive approach to challenging the wider social determinants of health, including the now widely documented social, political and economic factors known to mitigate against positive health outcomes (see for example Israel *et al.* 1994, Frohlich, Corin and Potvin 2001, Laverack 2001, Laverack and Wallerstein 2001, Frohlich *et al.* 2002, Laverack 2007, Wallerstein 2002, 2006, Abel and Frohlich 2012).

Notions of empowerment can be traced back to the social action theories and the feminist and social or grassroots movements of the 1960s and 1970s (Alinksy 1989, Anderson 1996, Kendall 1998, Wiggins 2011) and were heavily influenced by components of critical social theory and processes of collective consciousness raising and resistance (see Freire 1970, 1996, Habermas 1972, Giroux 1983). Many authors (see for example Campbell and MacPhail 2002, Wallerstein 2002, 2006, Delp, Brown and Domenzain 2005, Ataöv and Haider, 2006, Kerrigan *et al.* 2013) have drawn on these theories to highlight the importance of collective action and community participation in order to bring about political and social change in support of population health.

More recent uses of empowerment in health-related policy, however, have been strongly criticized for adopting an individualistic approach (see Grace 1991, Cook 2007, Baker 2008). Cook (2007), for instance, pointed to the popularity of empowerment in marketing and consumerist discourses, which create an illusion of 'free choice'. These individualistic uses of the term have been heavily criticized for failing to acknowledge and address broader relations of power that ultimately set limits to people's opportunities to 'choose' (Starkey 2003, Baker 2008). In her sharp criticism of empowerment, Grace (1991) argued that empowerment strategies simply reflect the ways in which individuals are constructed (and manipulated) as being health consumers capable of making 'empowered choices' but who remain subject to the control of health professionals and policymakers in decision-making processes (see also Bernstein *et al.* 1994). Consequently, people's needs are increasingly defined and shaped by consumerist and neoliberalist discourses that become disguised by utilizing concepts such as 'enabling' and 'empowering' (Grace 1991, Skelton 1994, Cook 2007, Baker 2008, Gill 2009). These individualistic uses of empowerment have thereby prompted a shift in the interpretation of the concept from one of collective action (with its central aim of effecting social change) to that of individual control and responsibility (Bernstein *et al.* 1994, Kendall 1998, Starkey 2003).

Despite these criticisms, concepts of empowerment remain evident in a number of successive UK government health policies (see for example DH 1992, 1999, 2004a and b, 2006, 2010a and b). Although these policies were developed under different British governments, these documents often uncritically link and conflate notions of empowerment with more individualized notions of 'user' and 'client' involvement and participation in health care (Poulton 1999, Morgan 2007, Martin and Finn 2011). These policies reflect some of the more recent organizational changes to the National Health Service (NHS) in the United Kingdom (see DH 2010a), which have sought to move the 'patient', 'client' or 'health consumer' to the centre of health policy (Thompson 2007, Martin and Finn 2011) and likewise stress the importance of empowering frontline staff in order to better serve the needs of patients.

> We will empower health professionals. Doctors and nurses must be able to use their professional judgement about what is right for patients. We will support this by giving frontline staff more control. Healthcare will be run from the bottom-up, with ownership and decision-making in the hands of professionals and patients. (DH 2010a, p. 1)

Rarely is empowerment defined in these documents, but nevertheless the concept is advocated as a positive approach to similarly engage patients, professionals and the public in health-related decision making (Ashworth, Longmate and Morrison 1992, Poulton 1999, Henwood *et al.* 2003, Morgan 2007).

Empowerment and young people

In recent times, and drawing in many ways on the principles enshrined in the United Nations Convention on the Rights of the Child (UNCRC) (UN Assembly 1989), this empowering participatory and partnership approach has been extended to policies focused on young people's health (see for example DH 2004a, 2010b, Department for Education and Skills [DfES]/ DH 2006, DCSF 2007). Examples of such participatory discourses can be found in various UK and wider international policy documents, including *Every Child Matters* (DfES 2003); *Choosing Health: Making Healthier Choices Easier* (DH 2004a); *National Service Framework for Children, Young People and Maternity Services* (DH 2004b); *National Healthy Schools Status: A Guide for Schools* (DfES/DH 2005); *Youth Matters: Next Steps* (DfES/DH 2006); *Aiming High for Young People: A Ten Year Strategy for Positive Activities* (Department for Children, Schools and Families [DCSF] 2007); *Healthy Lives, Brighter Futures – The Strategy for Children and Young People's Health* (DH/DCSF 2009); *Healthy Lives, Healthy People: Our Strategy for Public Health in England* (DH 2010b); *National Strategy for Young Australians* (Australian Government 2010) and *Making Health Services Adolescent Friendly* (WHO 2011a).

In recent Australian policy on young people's health, for example, the concept of empowerment features strongly in the government's national strategy to enhance young people's health and well-being. Specifically, empowerment is advocated as means through which young people will be given a 'voice and the opportunity to participate in on-going public debate on the issues that affect their lives' (Australian Government 2010, p. 21).

Likewise, in the United Kingdom, the government's *Aiming High* strategy set out a 'vision for empowerment' (DCSF 2007, p. 30). This included increasing young people's control over local spending; developing and prioritizing youth services that were responsive to young people's needs; and fostering a positive view of young people in society as a whole. The extension of the European Network for Health Promoting Schools (ENHPS) and development of the Healthy Schools Framework in the United Kingdom (DfES/DH 2005, ENHPS 2005) similarly prioritized the importance and development of responsive and sensitive health services for young people – specifically, highlighting the value of 'giving young people a voice' over matters of concern.

More recent UK health policy continues to prioritize concepts of empowerment (see DH 2010a and b). The public health white paper *Healthy Lives, Healthy People: Our Strategy for Public Health in England* (DH 2010b) advocated that a 'radical' shift in policy is needed to address 'lifestyle-driven health problems' through a 'new approach that empowers individuals to make healthy choices' (p. 2). As described in Chapter One, young people attract specific attention for their particular susceptibility to 'high-risk behaviours', with a focus on strengthening their self-esteem and confidence in order to empower them to 'choose' healthy lifestyles.

Although recent government policy in many Westernized nations has sought to empower young people by strengthening their self-esteem and confidence to make healthy choices, these policy documents do so through highlighting young people's responsibility in exercising the 'right' choices. These right choices typically refer to abstinence from risky health-related behaviours such as smoking, drinking alcohol, drug use, unsafe sex and unhealthy eating (see DH 2004a, DH 2010b). Young people's abilities to make the so-called right choice are then taken as examples and evidence of their 'empowerment' (Spencer, Maxwell and Aggleton 2008). These policy documents further discuss the concept of participation interchangeably and synonymously with empowerment, frequently highlighting a *need* to 'empower young people . . . to take greater control of their health and wellbeing by raising awareness of their risk taking behaviour' (DH/DCSF 2009, p. 45) – again reflecting more individualized notions of the concept.

By suggesting that young people's compliance with health promotion messages points to evidence of their empowerment, these policy documents appear to be largely set within a more predefined and protectionist risk-reduction framework. This approach exists in some contradiction with the original theoretical underpinnings of empowerment which, as set out in the previous chapter, typically foreground the importance of working from people's own concerns and which may well differ from official prescriptions on health. Although not seeking to simply 'explain away' some of the difficulties young people may encounter in terms of their health and health-related practices, these emergent contradictions in policy reveal a number of (unquestioned) assumptions and theoretical tensions concerning empowerment's relationship to young people's health.

First, and as some recent evidence suggests, official agendas drawing on the notion of empowerment may fail to resonate with young people's own health-related concerns and priorities (Ingham 2006, Percy-Smith 2006, 2007, Spencer 2008, Wills *et al.* 2008, Woodgate and Leach 2010) and crucially, take seriously the more positive and social aspects of young people's health and health-related practices (see Mitchell 1997, France 2000, Mitchell *et al.* 2001, Tulloch and Lupton 2003, Shoveller *et al.* 2004, 2010, van Exel, de Graaf and Brouwer 2006, Austen 2009, Lindsay 2009, Tutenges and Rod 2009, Harrison *et al.* 2011, Stead *et al.* 2011).

Second, this approach largely ignores how *choice* may be shaped and determined by social structures and contexts and, specifically, how *power* operates to facilitate and limit young people's so-called choices within any given context (Shoveller *et al.* 2004, 2010, Percy-Smith 2006, Gill 2007a, Baker 2008, Goldenberg *et al.* 2008, Evans and Davies 2010, Spencer, Doull and Shoveller 2012).

Third, this target-led approach to reducing young people's engagement with risky health behaviours therefore appears to define an empowerment agenda *for*, not *with*, young people. Consequently, by suggesting young people are in *need* of empowerment, such policies advocate a notion of empowerment that appears to be antithetical to many of the concept's original underpinnings by assuming young people want to be, and can be, empowered by others. Labonte (1989, 1993) highlighted this contradiction in the assertion that 'we cannot empower anybody, because to presume to do so strips people of their ability to choose. Groups and individuals can only empower and motivate themselves' (Labonte 1989, p. 24). Or, as Gomm (1993, p. 137) stated, 'To empower someone else implies something which is granted by someone more powerful to someone who is less powerful, a gift of power, made from a position of power'. Consequently, the current emphasis on empowerment, despite its suggested bottom-up approach, appears to *impose* an empowering agenda *on* young people.

Despite these tensions, empowerment continues to be presented as a 'good thing' in much health-related policy and health promotion practice.

Even within the academic literature, the positive relationship between empowerment and health appears to be taken for granted (see Curtis 1992, Essau 2004, Gordon and Turner 2004, Bishai, Mercer and Tapales 2005, Tengland 2007, 2008, Wilson *et al.* 2008). By doing so, this area of literature seems to depict a rather linear pathway from empowerment to positive health without offering a clear conceptualization of the word itself or indeed addressing the thorny theoretical tensions surrounding the concept's root word of *power*.

Conceptualizing empowerment

In light of these inconsistencies in use, I now turn to consider the various ways empowerment has been conceptualized in the broad field of health promotion. My aim here is to examine more thoroughly the meaning of empowerment by teasing out some of the crucial underpinning conceptual features of empowerment and how these conceptions may link to the various ways in which we understand the broad concept of health.

As suggested, efforts to conceptualize empowerment in the health-promotion literature highlight its polysemic nature (Eyben and Napier-Moore 2009). Definitions vary considerably in their emphasis on *individual* or *collective* responsibility for health, and empowerment as either a *process* or an *outcome* (Rappaport 1984, Zimmerman and Rappaport 1988, Gibson 1991, Israel *et al.* 1994, Rissel 1994, Schulz *et al.* 1995, Tones 2001, Wallerstein 2002, 2006). These distinctions can be linked back to the various definitions of health itself and the conceptual ambiguity that surrounds understanding what health means and how best to promote it.

Health can be understood in two broadly opposing ways (Duncan 2007). First, drawing on objectivism, health is often defined in physical terms and, specifically, as the absence of disease (Scadding 1988). Reflecting the biomedical paradigm, this more negative conceptualization of health draws attention to 'ill health' rather than the experience or achievement of positive health (Blaxter 2010). In contrast, a second definition of health is the 'foundation for achievement' (Seedhouse 2001) – reflecting a more positive conceptualization. Likewise, Antonovsky (1979) advocated the importance of thinking 'salutogenically' in order to capture the (positive) resources that may facilitate health – in contrast to a focus on the factors that prevent ill health.

Accordingly, health can be understood as holding multiple meanings and is constructed, experienced, embodied and enacted by individuals themselves (Lupton 2005, Blaxter 2010). The latter, more positive understandings of health are now evident in the growing body of literature that gives primacy to lay understandings of health (Lupton 1994, 2005) and can be seen to reflect more closely the WHO's (1946) well-known holistic definition of health as being 'a state of complete physical, mental and social well-being and not merely the absence of disease or infirmity'.

Based on these differing conceptualizations of health, a number of approaches to health promotion have been developed (see Tones and Tilford 2001, Naidoo and Wills 2009, Green and Tones 2010). Although the nature and purpose of health promotion has itself been subject to much debate (see Duncan 2004), broadly defined, these different approaches include the biomedical approach based on the prevention of disease, behaviour change approaches that encourage people to take up health-enhancing behaviours (see Ajzen and Fishbein 1980, Prochaska and DiClemente 1984), educational approaches that seek to provide individuals with knowledge and skills to make informed decisions about their health (see Tones and Tilford 2001) and social change approaches that seek to change policy and socio-economic environments to facilitate healthy choices (Milio 1986, Naidoo and Wills 2009). As described, empowerment-based approaches became increasingly popular within health promotion and public health following a number of WHO statements on health (WHO 1977, 1986, 2005). These empowerment-based approaches were further supported by the widespread uptake of the WHO's definition of health promotion as 'the process of enabling people to increase control over and improve their health' (WHO 1986, p. 1) – capturing both the individual and political dimensions of health.

Many authors take the WHO definition of health promotion as a starting point for conceptualizing empowerment and subsequently prioritize concepts of control within their various definitions of empowerment. Gibson (1991, p. 359), for example, defined empowerment as 'a social process of recognizing, promoting and enhancing people's abilities to meet their own needs, solve their own problems and mobilize the necessary resources in order to feel in control of their lives'. Similarly, in an earlier definition, Rappaport (1984) defined empowerment as 'the mechanism by which people, organizations and communities gain mastery over their lives' (p. 1). Wallerstein's (2002) definition of empowerment suggests a more dynamic interpretation, capturing the multilayered nature of the concept as being 'a social action process by which individuals, communities and organizations gain mastery over their lives in the context of changing their social and political environment to improve equity and quality of life' (p. 73).

These varying definitions capture the idea that empowerment is something developed and gained by people themselves, rather than granted or given by others, and is therefore often discussed as a 'bottom-up' (in contrast to a 'top-down') strategy for health promotion (see Labonte 1989, Tones 1998a and b, Laverack 2009).

Other more recent definitions of empowerment prioritize the concept of power (Thompson 2007, McDaid 2010, Spencer 2013a). Laverack (2009, p. xi) maintained that 'empowerment, the means to attaining power, is a process of capacity building, with the goal of bringing about social and political change in favour of the individuals, groups and communities seeking more control'. Cook (2007) defined empowerment as 'acquiring power for oneself' (p. 7). Thompson (2007) similarly linked the concept of power to empowerment as 'helping people gain greater control over their lives and circumstances' (p. 21) at three different levels of power – personal, cultural, and structural. These definitions again highlight the importance of control but extend their conceptualization of empowerment to encompass how a stronger understanding of power can help practitioners facilitate the necessary (social) conditions for empowerment at both individual and community levels.

Much of the health promotion literature on empowerment draws an important distinction between *psychological* or individual empowerment and *community* or collective forms of empowerment (Rissel 1994, Tones and Tilford 2001, Manojlovich 2007, Laverack 2009). Psychological empowerment links most closely to social psychology theories, including Bandura's (1977, 1982) social learning theory and Rotter's (1966) locus of control model. This (individual) notion of empowerment is often associated with the development of an individual's self-efficacy and enhancing self-esteem and perceptions of personal control as being the first 'stage' of empowerment (Rappaport 1984, Zimmerman 1990, 1995, Kuokkanen and Leino-Kilpi 2001, Bradbury-Jones, Sambrook and Irvine 2008, Nation *et al.* 2008, Morton and Montgomery 2011). Tones (1998a and b) maintained that such psychological or self-empowerment can occur through education, which facilitates the development of personal skills and critical thinking (see also Zimmerman 1990, 1995). This understanding prioritizes the *process* of empowerment through highlighting a number of personal attributes individuals can develop in order to enhance their sense of empowerment (or *power within*). This interpretation of empowerment closely reflects many current (individualistic) uses of empowerment in health policy but says little about whether empowerment, once reached, is maintained or may indeed *shift* according to context.

Community or collective forms of empowerment, on the other hand, involve the mobilization of individuals into communities to take action against the disempowering effects of the sociopolitical environment (Israel *et al.* 1994, Rissel 1994, Wallerstein 2002, Williams and Labonte 2007, Laverack 2009, Wiggins 2011). Community empowerment approaches draw variously on community participation and development perspectives (Rifkin 1990, Labonte 1996), Putnam's (1993, 1995) notion of 'social capital'[1] (see Briggs 2010 for an example) and Paulo Freire's (1970) discussion of *conscientização* or critical consciousness raising (see Campbell and MacPhail 2002, Prins 2008, Mohajer and Earnest 2009, 2010 for some examples). These approaches further seek to better address and tackle the dynamic interplay and relationship between social structure and individual agency (Frohlich *et al.* 2002, Williams 2003, Abel 2008, Rütten and Gelius 2011, Abel and Frohlich 2012). An important prerequisite within these interpretations is that by identifying challenges to their health (and the potential solutions to such challenges) communities themselves can define and control their own health-related agendas (Rissel 1994, Laverack 2007,

2009, Wiggins 2011). According to such perspectives, the key *outcome* of empowerment is to bring about social change to redress the disempowering conditions of the social context through, for example, gaining greater access to the resources that people themselves identify as being necessary to bring about change. This understanding can thus be seen to more closely reflect the WHO's use and interpretation of health promotion and broader calls within public health to address wider health and social inequalities (Laverack 2004, Wiggins 2011, Abel and Frohlich 2012).

Within much of the health promotion literature, empowerment is further depicted as a rather linear continuum from individual to collective empowerment (Williams and Labonte 2007, Pearrow and Pollack 2009) and from a position of powerlessness to being powerful. This continuum suggests that individuals first need to empower themselves (most usually through increases to self-esteem and confidence) before coming together as a group of empowered individuals to form (a more powerful) empowered collective (see for example Tones and Tilford 2001, Laverack 2007). This continuum has a tendency to suggest empowerment is a rather stable concept (Nation *et al.* 2008) and fails to acknowledge the possibility of more variable and indeterminate outcomes arising from processes of empowerment, or indeed how empowerment may shift in and between different contexts (see for example Holland *et al.* 2004). In the chapters that follow, I reveal how these underlying contradictions and inconsistencies in use may play out in the realm of young people's health – offering both possibilities for, and limitations of, empowerment.

Conclusion

In this chapter I have sought to highlight some of the diverse meanings and uses of empowerment across a range of literatures and areas of practice. In particular, the chapter has illustrated the ways in which the concept has been taken up in recent health-related policy to encourage individuals to take responsibility for their health and adopt expert-defined healthy behaviours. The chapter has also charted some of the origins of the concept and, specifically, the increasing use and popularity of empowerment in the broad field of health promotion.

Within the health promotion literature, definitions of empowerment vary considerably in their emphasis on *individual* or *collective* notions of empowerment; the former with its origins in theories from social psychology, and the latter more firmly placed within critical social theory and specifically, Freirean notions of critical consciousness raising. The health promotion literature also makes an important distinction between processes and outcomes of empowerment and by doing so, seems to suggest a rather linear pathway from empowerment to positive health.

In this chapter I have further argued that much of the literature on young people's health to date continues to advocate empowerment (often used interchangeably with the concept of participation) without clear conceptualization of the word itself, or indeed its root word – *power*, an understanding of which may offer different possibilities for understanding empowerment. In the chapter that follows, I consider how a full-fledged engagement with differing concepts of power may help to advance the conceptualization of empowerment and, thus better explain the concept's relationship to, and relevance for, young people's health.

3 Power, empowerment and young people

This chapter takes up the discussion on power to help advance the conceptualization of empowerment and better explain the concept's relationship to, and relevance for, young people's health. The chapter is in two main parts. First, I examine a number of perspectives on power (*power to, power within, power over, power through*) and consider their implications for understanding the related concept of empowerment. The aim of this analysis is to bring to the fore some of the unquestioned assumptions and theoretical tensions surrounding current uses of empowerment. Concepts of resistance and forms of critical consciousness raising are also discussed for their relevance to understanding the concept of empowerment. The discussion on power concludes by drawing on a particular perspective of power offered by Steven Lukes (1974, 2005). Lukes's tripartite perspective of power is considered especially appropriate for furthering an understanding of the concept of empowerment since it provides a framework that integrates the multiple ways power has been conceptualized and operates at individual, structural and ideological levels.

Drawing on Lukes's framework of power, in the second part of this chapter I draw together some of the recent empirical evidence to investigate the purported relationship between empowerment, young people and health. My aim here is to consider the possibilities for (and limitations of) empowerment as given in the current literature by engaging with a full-fledged theorization of power. Here, I put forward two key arguments. First, by drawing on evidence of young people's 'resistance' to dominant health promotion messages, the widely held assumption that empowerment straightforwardly translates into positive health outcomes is questioned. Second, the discussion illustrates how current uses of empowerment may unwittingly reinforce, rather than shift, existing power relations – with important implications for young people's health and opportunities for health promotion.

Theorizing power

Concepts of power are central to understanding the term *empowerment* (Ryles 1999, Lincoln *et al.* 2002, Thompson 2007, Laverack 2009). Laverack

(2009) defined empowerment as the act of attaining power and is evident in people's abilities to exercise choice in their lives. Broadly defined, power is often conceptualized as the capacity or agency to act – *power to;*[1] personal mastery and control – *power within;*[2] exert control over others – *power-over;*[3] and *power through,*[4] highlighting more ideological forms of power and the micropolitics of power operating through discursive practices. Power is further discussed in terms of 'fixed' or 'zero-sum' models whereby the amount of power in society is seen as constant so that if one group accumulates power it does so at the expense of another (for example, pluralist[5] perspectives). In contrast, 'variable-sum' models point to different and changing 'levels' of power, which may be held by certain social (dominant) groups (for example, structuralist perspectives) or dispersed within and between social groups and contexts (for example, Foucauldian perspectives).

Whilst originating in different schools of thought, these interpretations of power illustrate some of the multiple and various ways in which power may operate. My intention here is not to undertake the difficult (and perhaps elusive) task of detailing all contributions made to date but instead to synthesize some of the major contributions to the theorization of power. The discussion that follows therefore considers these contributions in the following ways: *power to and power within, power over, and power through.* The aim of this analysis is to uncover some of the rarely addressed thorny theoretical tensions and operational challenges surrounding current conceptions of empowerment. These tensions are then further interrogated and illustrated by drawing on the literature on young people, empowerment and health in the final part of this chapter.

Power to and power within

A *power to* understanding of the concept captures the importance of an individual's ability to act or influence others (Hearn 2012) and links closely with agency perspectives of power (see for example Archer 1988, McNay 2000, 2003, Lovell 2003, Clegg 2006, Campbell 2009, Hearn 2012). Wrong (2002, p. 2), for example, defined power as being 'the capacity of some persons to produce intended and foreseen affects on others' – suggesting an element of intentionality on behalf of the individual. This implied use of intentionality can be traced back to some early philosophical perspectives such as those provided by Machiavelli (1958 [original 1517]). For Machiavelli, power was defined as a strategic and operational tool that could be, and should be, used for one's own interest, specifically, foregrounding an individual's capacity to act and achieve his or her own ends. Likewise, although also reflecting a *power over* conceptualization, Dahl's 'agency model of power' exemplifies a *power to* perspective and draws attention to the forms of power operating within decision-making processes whereby 'A has power over B to the extent that he can get B to do something B would not otherwise do' (Dahl 1957, p. 203).

These *power to* interpretations of the concept point to a notion of empowerment that links to the development of an individual's ability to enact decision-making. Although not always explicitly noted in the literature, these perspectives can be seen in much of the health promotion literature emphasizing those more individual forms of empowerment that take a specific focus on developing an individual's self-esteem and self-efficacy (see for example, Tones 1998a, Zimmerman 1990, 1995). Drawing on theories from social psychology, these individualistic uses of empowerment also capture a dispositional or *power within* interpretation, whereby an individual can develop and gain a sense of control and personal mastery linked to the development of a number of personal attributes (Rappaport 1984, Rowlands 1998, Zimmerman 1990). More recent literature has begun to consider the role and significance of these affective dimensions as triggering an individual's subjective feelings of power or *power within* to bring about (social) change (see for example, Evans, Riley and Shankar 2010, Gavey 2012).

These more individualized conceptions, however, have been heavily criticized for downplaying the significance of structural forms of power; the latter a firm feature within many theories of power originating from sociology and political science – reflecting *power over* conceptualizations.

Power over

Power over interpretations of the concept highlight various forms of domination. Reflecting a consensus perspective, Parsons (1967) offered a variable-sum model of power to suggest domination as a social good. For Parsons, power was understood as being a positive and productive social resource for the achievement of agreed social goals. Any inequitable distribution of *power over* is therefore legitimized as a functional prerequisite for the effective operation and maintenance of the social order. Such an interpretation appears to negate any need for empowerment and arguably renders the concept redundant since power operates and is exercised for the benefit of a meritocratic social order. Inevitably conflict theorists, including those working within various strands of Marxism and feminism, have attacked this productive perspective of power and point to experiences of oppression and exploitation whereby power is held by a ruling minority and exercised *over* the majority.

Traditional Marxist perspectives on power, for example, foreground varying forms of economic and capitalist *power over* interpretations (see Miliband 1969, Althusser 1971, Poulantzas 1976). Power is exercised over the majority by, and in the (economic) interests of, a ruling class minority. Accordingly, power is held by the owners of the means of production, which in turn is supported and perpetuated by the State and its governing institutions. As a consequence, economic power yields political power (see Miliband 1969) and ideological power (see Althusser 1971) whereby acceptance of, and compliance with, the ruling dominant ideology is maintained through society's structures and institutions. For Marxists, *praxis*[6] is the site for emancipatory practice and revolution and points to a notion of empowerment that would ultimately result in the redistribution of economic power.

Likewise, some strands of traditional feminist perspectives offer a *power over* interpretation. However, gender, rather than class or economic relations, is the central point of analysis and specifically, an examination of men's dominance *over* women. Liberal feminism, for example, presents a fixed-sum perspective, defining power as a resource to be redistributed through society's structures and institutions more equally between men and women (see Mill 1970 and Okin 1989). Through the collective and political mobilization of women, challenges to prevailing male dominated economic and political systems can be made. The resulting redistribution of power and subsequent empowerment of women would be thus evidenced in examples of equal opportunities and access to social positions for both men and women.

Radical feminists similarly conceptualize power as domination. This interpretation of power is relational, emphasizing male domination and women's subordination. However, radical feminism heavily emphasizes the system of patriarchy, in contrast to capitalism (cf. Marxist feminism), as the source of women's oppression. Mackinnon (1987) argued that the system of patriarchy creates gender divisions and subsequently defines men as powerful and women as powerless. According to these perspectives, patriarchal constructions of masculinity and femininity not only reify men's domination, but also lead to the universal acceptance of patriarchy, thereby exposing ideological, as opposed to structural, forms of power. This form of analysis, however, has been heavily criticized for promoting traditional gender binaries by suggesting a zero-sum model of power whereby any evidence of women's empowerment would seem to imply men's 'disempowerment'. Whilst presenting possibilities for young women's empowerment, this perspective therefore makes it difficult to consider the implications and possibilities for young men's empowerment. This zero-sum interpretation of power does, however, raise an important question; namely, whether the empowerment of one group results in the disempowerment of another.

A further *power over* perspective particularly relevant to understanding the concept of empowerment as it relates to young people is that offered by generational perspectives. Drawing on Mannheim's (1952) concept of 'generation' as 'a socially constructed system of relationships amongst social positions' (Alanen 2001, p. 12), contributions to the sociology of generations literatures have sought to examine the structuring principles and effects of age that work alongside other forms of social organization such as those linked to class position, gender and ethnicity (Pilcher 1994, James and Prout 1997, Alanen and Mayall 2001, Mayall 2002). The concept of generation points to the common social location people occupy by virtue of experiencing the same social location and reveals how some of the inequities and inequalities people experience are a consequence of being defined on the basis of age. Drawing on Mannheim's generational perspective, a now growing body of literature from within the sociology of childhood[7] has highlighted the various ways in which adults exercise *power over* children and young people (James and Prout 1997, Mayall 2002, Jenks 2005, Mannion 2007, Bjerke 2011).

Whilst Mannheim's notion of generation reflects a *power over* interpretation, with a specific focus on an individual's or group's location in the social structure, this perspective also highlights ideological features, as assumptions linked to the social category of age are essentialized as being part of the natural order of society. Any empowerment stemming from a generational perspective would therefore necessitate an examination of, and challenge to, the ways in which the social (rather than biological) category of age not only produces and reproduces structural inequities and inequalities, but also the *normative* assumptions linked to understandings of age – thereby indicating the significance of ideological perspectives of power that work along with (and through) *power to* and *power over* conceptualizations.

Power through

A *power through* conceptualization highlights the ways in which power comes to define and shape dominant ideas, norms and values. Gramsci (1971) made a conceptual distinction between an understanding of power as domination or *power over* (which is linked to the State) and that of the exercise of hegemony, which serves to shape social consensus and legitimate dominant rule or *power through* ideology. According to Gramsci, hegemony is produced and maintained through producing the active consent of a dominated majority. Through the acceptance and naturalization of cultural practices, broad social consensus is achieved as dominant interests are embraced, rather than imposed, by society. However, whilst hegemony is embraced it can be also resisted and mediated through everyday counterhegemonic practices. Indeed, for the dominant ideology to prevail, concessions to competing ideologies and interests are necessary and often granted. Consequently, concessions on secondary issues are made to maintain support for dominant interests and illustrate how any resistance or counterhegemony remains set *within* the dominant hegemony.

Drawing on Gramsci's concept of hegemony, proponents of the dominant ideology thesis (Abercrombie, Hill and Turner 1980; see also Miliband 1969, Althusser 1971, Habermas 1972) also point to ideological forms of *power through* whereby dominant interests are naturalized and uncritically accepted as the normal order of society. Althusser's (1971) early analysis of the Ideological State Apparatus outlined the necessary conditions for the reproduction of the economic system according to class interests. However, Abercrombie, Hill and Turner (1980) maintained that ideology can be produced independently of class interests and achieves its effects by constructing and placing individuals as particular subjects within the social system but, at the same time, conceals their capacity and roles as *agents* within that structure.

Similarly, but from a poststructuralist perspective, Scott (1990) identified ideological dimensions of power in his distinction between a 'public transcript' (which reflects the open ideology of the powerful), and a 'hidden transcript'. The hidden transcript is a site for resistance against the public transcript as oppositional ideas and practices of marginalized groups challenge the nature of the public transcript.

More recent poststructuralist perspectives of power, often informed by the extensive work of Michel Foucault (1980, 1988, 1990) on power/ knowledge, also indicate *power through* interpretations (see also Bourdieu 1990, 1991, 1993). For Foucault, power was not fixed but was constantly shifting, meeting points of resistance to produce and reproduce discourse (Foucault 1980). Similar to Parsons' productive and facilitative interpretation of power, Foucault unpicked the micropolitics of power that operate through discourse, defining and producing truth claims that are subsequently accepted and adopted as legitimate and normalized frameworks of knowledge. Disciplinary power thereby ensues as normalized patterns of behaviour are produced to regulate individuals and populations (Foucault 1988, 1991, Lupton 1995, 2013, Ryles 1999). Foucault's notion of 'governmentality' dominates political power and acts as a form of social regulation and control. Consequently, 'official' guidelines, advice and methods of surveillance produce conformity and comparison to 'expert' norms (Lupton 1995, 2013).

More recent feminist perspectives drawing on Foucault have emphasized the micropolitics and more relational aspects and effects of gendered disciplinary power (Bordo 1988, Bartky 1990, Gill 2007a and b, 2008). Dietary practices, beauty rituals and reproductive technologies offer examples of women's self-surveillance and obedience to gendered disciplinary practices (see Bartky 1990, Lazar 2011). Consequently, women exercise disciplinary practices on themselves in support of men's interests that further serve to create and sustain a 'normative femininity' (Bartky 1990, Gill 2008).

Within public health, examples of these forms of disciplinary power or *power through* perspectives are evidenced in the increasing methods of health surveillance and screening. Lupton (1995, 1999a and b, 2013) highlighted how these methods of surveillance effectively serve to define, measure and regulate individual behaviour through a notion of an ideal or optimal health. Examples of these processes can be seen in those areas of health education and promotion that aim to encourage people to adopt healthy lifestyles and change and regulate their behaviour according to 'expert' systems of knowledge (Lupton 1995, 1999a and b, 2013, Duff 2003, Crawford 2004, Armstrong and Murphy 2011). Such forms of disciplinary power can be further seen in the UK government policy *Choosing Health* (Department of Health [DH] 2004a) – the title itself implicitly suggesting that individuals themselves make the decision to be healthy.

Based on expert knowledge and advice, this policy points to the ways in which people themselves can actively *choose* health through, for example, eating a balanced diet, taking regular exercise, giving up smoking and moderating their consumption of alcohol.

In response to these forms of disciplinary power, the self-regulating health-conscious individual therefore adopts (and even self-chooses) to govern and (self-)regulate his or her own behaviours in line with accepted and 'normal' patterns of healthy behaviour (Lupton 1995, 2013, Armstrong and Murphy 2011). This reflexive and self-regulating individual gives rise to what Foucault termed the 'technologies of the self' whereby individuals themselves actively seek expert knowledge in the pursuit of the idealized self (Foucault 1988). However, these forms of disciplinary power are not imposed without resistance – indeed, it is this resistance that continues to produce and reproduce power. Resistance is therefore an instrument and effect of power; without resistance there would be no power (Clegg 1998). An understanding of power as resistance is therefore central to understanding the possibilities for empowerment based on any *power through* conceptualization.

Power as resistance

Clegg's (1998) analysis of power indicates the importance of resistance to understanding the concept of power. Based on three distinct but interconnecting circuits – episodic, dispositional and facilitative – Clegg saw power not as something people hold or possess but instead as an unstable and shifting phenomenon moving through distinct systems and circuits of power, meeting points of resistance. Power is therefore understood as a dynamic and relational concept, moving between and within structure and agency (cf. Giddens 1987, 1991).[8] In agreement with Foucault, Clegg argued that resistance is itself power, which is at its most pervasive when it is reified. The reification of power occurs when power is considered to be 'real, solid and material' (Clegg 1998, p. 207), a process which frequently occurs in the face of resistance.

Drawing upon Clegg and Foucault's work, any notion of empowerment informed by this interpretation of power must therefore examine the possibilities for resistance that are present within a particular context. However, the potential for such resistance to reinforce, rather than challenge, existing power relations has been empirically demonstrated in earlier youth subcultural literatures (see Hall and Jefferson 1976, Willis 1977, McRobbie 1978) and links to Gramsci's suggestion that any counter-hegemonic processes themselves are usually bounded by the parameters of the dominant hegemony (see also Allen 2003a and b, and Gill 2008 from a poststructuralist perspective). Consequently, resistance may become a site of social *reproduction* rather than *transformation* – thereby pointing to the relevance of methods of critical pedagogy and forms of consciousness raising (see Freire 1970, 1996, Habermas 1972, Giroux 1983), which seek to generate critical awareness of the processes of social and cultural reproduction to bring about social change.

Critical consciousness raising

Freire's (1970, 1996) critical pedagogy outlines an approach to facilitating *conscientização* or critical consciousness raising (CCR), amongst oppressed groups with the purported effect of challenging and transforming disempowering contexts. The process of CCR aims to facilitate the unity of individuals who then collectively recognize the commonalty of their disempowered positions in order to bring about social change. Freire argued that in order for people to be liberated from oppression, 'people must first critically recognize its causes' (Freire 1996, p. 29). The greatest challenge to such liberation is the internalization and uncritical acceptance of oppression – thereby drawing attention to the significance of Clegg's argument regarding the reification of power.

For Freire, the Marxian concept of *praxis* is the means through which power can be reified to bring about social change. Praxis is achieved through CCR and a cycle of theory, reflection and action, which helps people recognize their internalization and acceptance of their own oppression (Freire 1970). Similar to Habermas's (1970) notion of therapeutic dialogue and theory of communicative action,[9] Freire's discussion of CCR highlights the importance of educators to initiate a critical dialogue based upon mutual respect and cooperation with groups and individuals. This approach now appears as a key component of many collective approaches to empowerment (see for example Wallerstein and Bernstein 1988, 1994, Wallerstein and Sanchez-Merki 1994, Hage and Lorensen 2005, Wallerstein, Sanchez-Merki and Velarde 2005, Fletcher 2006, Mohajer and Earnest 2009, 2010).

Freire's approach, however, has been criticized on a number of grounds. First, those in a position to facilitate the process of CCR (such as educators) may themselves be biased toward a particular perspective – thereby steering people's views accordingly (Macedo 1995). Consequently, one form of cultural bias is merely replaced by another because those in more powerful positions are more able to assert their version of 'truth' (Howe 1994, Gillman 1996, Hui and Stickley 2007). This critique points to a further poststructuralist argument, which challenges the (realist) suggestion that it is possible to identify accepted 'truths'.

Moreover, although CCR may initiate resistance to particular ideological interpretations of power, Freire said little about the way in which such resistance is then defined and appropriated within the context of everyday action – not just by those displaying such resistance but also by those for whom such resistance is challenging, which may ultimately set limits to any related empowerment. As previously suggested, the possibility that young people's resistance could be reframed as evidence of their unruliness and deviance (rather than their empowerment) reveals how any responses to forms of CCR may also support processes of social reproduction, rather than transformation – a crucial point further examined and exemplified in Part Two of the book.

The chapter thus far has examined various interpretations of power and how they might begin to help inform an understanding of empowerment based on an underpinning *power to*, *power over* and *power through* conceptualization. By doing so, I have sought to underscore the importance of understanding related conceptions of power, including forms of resistance and methods of critical consciousness raising as a means to potentially shift dominant power relations. I now conclude this discussion on power by drawing on a particular perspective of power offered by Steven Lukes (2005). Lukes's three-dimensional analysis of power provides a framework that integrates the multiple ways in which power may operate at individual, structural and ideological levels. This form of analysis is considered especially appropriate for examining the related concept of empowerment since it draws together some of the perspectives of power outlined previously and, by doing so, helps to expose some further theoretical tensions within existing uses and conceptualizations of empowerment from various interpretations of power. These emerging tensions are then examined more fully in relation to the empirical literature on empowerment, young people and health in the concluding section of this chapter.

Steven Lukes's radical view of power

Lukes's (2005) radical view of power[10] highlights three dimensions of power that synthesize the individual, structural and ideological relations of influence over people's lives – capturing the diverse ways power has been understood in terms of *power to, power over* and *power through* conceptualizations. At the individual level, Lukes's first dimension exemplifies the power that is evident in open conflicts of interest and decision-making and reflects a *power to* understanding. However, according to Lukes, evidence of the operation of power at this level fails to acknowledge the power that may restrict issues from reaching open debate, giving rise to what Lukes coined the second dimension of power, which draws on Bachrach and Baratz's (1962) critique of Dahl's one-dimensional and agency model of power. This second dimension refers to nonobservable conflicts and represents the power of those who set and control the decision-making agenda and consequently hold *power over* preventing issues from reaching mainstream discussion.

Lukes's third dimension of power is explicitly ideological in nature and represents the power that effectively shapes desires and wishes reflecting those *power through* interpretations similar to Foucault's (1980, 1990) notion of disciplinary power, Marxian notions of false consciousness (Marx and Engels 1959), Althusser's (1971) notion of ideological state apparatus, and Gramsci's (1971) concept of hegemony. Crucially, Lukes's third dimension of power draws important attention to processes of social and cultural reproduction that typically support dominant knowledge systems and interests. As a consequence, dominant frameworks of understanding and practice are legitimized, becoming accepted as part of the natural social order.

Whilst Lukes's first and second dimensions of power point to possibilities for young people's empowerment to exercise decision-making and potentially shape health-related agendas, it is important to acknowledge some limitations to this framework and, specifically, how the third dimension of power may present a number of paradoxes for understanding empowerment. Arguably, any definition of empowerment based on Lukes's third dimension of power would seem to necessitate an exploration and understanding of what might be young people's 'real' interests. However, just as criticisms have been made of Freire's CCR, so it seems somewhat problematic to consider what young people's 'real' interests might be, given the possible effects of ideology in potentially shaping such interests. This raises epistemological issues concerning the nature of truth and knowledge and highlights the significance of those interpretations of power that work *through* knowledge structures and discourses (cf. Foucault and Bourdieu) and further, how an understanding of resistance may offer possibilities to shift *power through* dominant frameworks of knowing. Indeed, in line with his more recent contribution, Lukes himself has acknowledged these criticisms – highlighting too the relevance of understanding power as a more productive, dynamic and potentially transformative concept (see Lukes 2005, Swartz 2007).

Power, empowerment and young people

Drawing on this tripartite framework of power (*power to, power over, power through*), I now conclude this chapter on power by bringing together recent empirical evidence that suggests some possible links between empowerment and young people's health. This final section illustrates how different uses of empowerment in the literature on young people and health can be linked to varying interpretations of power. By engaging with a full-fledged theorization of power, my aim here is to expose some further theoretical tensions surrounding current uses of (and identify some key prerequisites for) empowerment in relation to young people's health – thereby providing the impetus for further empirical enquiry on empowerment, young people and health (the focus of Part Two of the book).

Power within or power to? Individualistic approaches to young people's empowerment

As I have argued previously, much of the existing literature on empowerment, young people and health appears to promote and align with a more individualistic and *power to* interpretation of the concept. As described in Chapter Two, this individualistic approach to empowerment is a feature of much recent health-related policy with a specific focus on increasing young people's *power within* through the development of their self-esteem, confidence and knowledge of health risks associated with particular health behaviours (see DH 2004a, 2010b, Wight and Dixon 2004, Wild *et al.* 2004, Pearson 2006, Nation *et al.* 2008). Evidence that suggests a lack of self-esteem is associated with negative health-related behaviours (see Emler 2001, Jayakody *et al.* 2005, Morton and Montgomery 2011) arguably supports the relevance of this individualistic and *power to* understanding of empowerment to the promotion of young people's health.

By measuring increases in young people's health-related knowledge, self-esteem, attitudinal and behavioural change (see for example Hawton *et al.* 2002, Reininger *et al.* 2003, Wild *et al.* 2004, Busseri, Willoughby and Chalmers 2007), this area of literature frequently suggests that increases in knowledge or changes to behaviour can be taken as evidence of young people's 'empowerment' (Tisdall and Davis 2004, Wight and Dixon 2004). In many ways, these highly individualistic approaches to empowerment thus become relatively indistinguishable from more traditional health promotion models of behaviour change (Duncan and Cribb 1996) and thus raise a number of difficulties for understanding the concept's relationship to young people's health.

First, based largely on a narrow biomedical definition of health, these individualistic approaches uncritically assume that increases in health-related knowledge readily translate into positive health behaviours. This simplistic linkage fails to acknowledge the now extensive body of literature that indicates the limited successes of individualistic behavioural change approaches (see Webb and Sheeran 2006, Shepherd *et al.* 2010, Spencer, Doull and Shoveller 2012). Hoppe *et al.* (2004) demonstrated that in the United States young people were well informed of health risks associated with unprotected sex but that this knowledge in itself was not associated with changes in individual behaviour – a finding widely echoed elsewhere in the literature on young people's health (see Skidmore and Hayter 2000, Denscombe 2001a and b, Stone and Ingham 2002, Stjerna, Lauritzen and Tillgren 2004, Ingham 2006, Katainen 2006).

Second, these individualistic approaches fail to engage with evidence demonstrating young people's active *choice* to engage in practices that adults and health professionals may consider as being harmful or risky to health (see for example Denscombe 2001a, Katainen 2006, Abbott and Dalla 2008). As previously described, this body of research draws important attention to the ways in which pleasure, choice and autonomy often guide young people's health-related practices (Green, Mitchell and Bunton 2000, Denscombe 2000, 2001a and b, Ingham 2005, Hunt, Evans and Kares 2007, Pilkington 2007, Spencer 2008, Austen 2009, Griffin *et al.* 2009, Harrison *et al.* 2011, Nelson, MacDonald and Abbott 2012).

In research with young people, these more positive dimensions have been found to include 'having fun' (van Exel, de Graaf and Brouwer 2006, Lindsay 2009, Tutenges and Rod 2009), supporting the development of a sense of identity (Denscombe 2001b, Nichter *et al.* 2006, Haines, Poland and Johnson 2009, Stead *et al.* 2011) and promoting peer acceptance (Denscombe 2000, Stead *et al.* 2011). Findings from other research with young people in Europe and Canada highlight how engaging in collective health-related practices may support forms of cultural and symbolic capital linked to the expression of particular styles and tastes (Järvinen and Gundelach 2007, Haines, Poland and Johnson 2009), thereby enabling young people to better negotiate and reach valued social positions (see also Room and Sato 2002, Stead *et al.* 2011).

Such evidence challenges findings demonstrating that risky behaviours are indicators of young people's low self-esteem (Hawton *et al.* 2002, Wild *et al.* 2004, Jayakody *et al.* 2005) or as a consequence of their 'disempowerment'. Findings from this area of research may in fact indicate that resisting dominant health advice (often in full knowledge of the risks involved) may directly increase levels of autonomy and empowerment for some young people (West and Sweeting 1997, McGee and Williams 2000, Denscombe 2001a, Turner and Gordon 2004, Katainen 2006). This body of evidence therefore raises some important and crucial questions about whether empowerment (based on a *power to* conceptualization) results in positive health outcomes as defined by official health discourse. However, if not, it seems somewhat problematic for the concept to remain a central goal of health promotion.

Third, this area of the literature assumes that young people will be simply empowered through increases in knowledge without addressing wider concerns for, and access to, material resources and services that enable them to act on such knowledge (Goldenberg *et al.* 2008, Shoveller *et al.* 2010). These approaches therefore seem to equate perceived control with actual control, thereby ignoring structural forms of power (or *power over* interpretations) which position some young people in disempowering or 'unhealthy' contexts. Consequently, *power to* interpretations could be seen to contribute to the reproduction of asymmetrical power relations through promoting an illusionary perception of control (see also Gill 2008).

Recent research with young people in the USA and Canada, for example, demonstrates some of the limits and barriers to exercising health-related choices (Croll, Neumark-Sztainer and Story 2001, Goldenberg *et al.* 2008, Shoveller *et al.* 2010). Likewise, Bauer, Yang and Austin (2004) found that young people's 'choice' to eat healthy foods was significantly limited by the cost and availability of such foods both inside and outside of school. Consequently, young people were found to have few options but to consume foods deemed unhealthy – a finding reiterated in other research on young people's health (see Story, Neumark-Sztainer and French 2002, Maes and Livens 2003, Shoveller *et al.* 2004).

Evidence of this kind not only troubles the notion of 'choice' (Baker 2008, Spencer, Doull and Shoveller 2012) but also prompts serious concern with processes of empowerment and that of raising young people's expectations. As Gallagher and Burden (1994) argued, it would appear highly problematic and even unethical to 'encourage people that they ought to do something if they do not have the capacity to do so' (p. 56). Consequently, some authors have highlighted how empowerment may inadvertently raise awareness of people's 'powerlessness' to change the oppressive nature of their socioeconomic environments, with 'disempowering' consequences (Wallerstein and Bernstein 1994, McDaid 2010).

Finally, such evidence further exemplifies a key argument I raised at the outset of this chapter – namely, that current uses of the concept of empowerment have moved away from the concept's original theoretical underpinnings by *imposing* a framework of empowerment on young people. This more top-down approach fails to question whether young people themselves would identify empowerment as a potential means to promote their health – a point not taken up in the current literature.

Power with or power over? Participatory and collective approaches to young people's empowerment

An increasing part of the literature on empowerment and young people's health draws on concepts of participation and specifically, Freire's notion of CCR (see for example Campbell and MacPhail 2002, Jennings *et al.* 2006, Mohajer and Earnest 2009, 2010). These more collective approaches seek to develop young people's abilities to exercise *power over* their own lives through critical reflection on how power may operate to marginalize their views and now widely feature in broader international literatures examining varying examples of youth activism (see Gordon 2007, Butler and Princeswal 2010, Coe *et al.* 2012).

As previously suggested, in many Westernized nations, recent health-related policy often prioritizing notions of participation (frequently discussed interchangeably with the concept of empowerment) as a means to encourage young people's involvement in shaping health-related priorities (see for example Department for Children, Schools and Families 2007, DH 2010b, Australian Government 2010, WHO 2011a). In line with this policy emphasis, there are now many empirical examples of efforts to work in partnership with young people and, specifically, to encourage young people's participation in shaping and developing local services and policy to support their health (Dalrymple 2001, Cavet and Sloper 2004, Barber 2007, Milbourne 2009). Often drawing on participatory action research techniques (see Rindner 2002, Perrons and Skyers 2003, Ataöv and Haider 2006, Jennings *et al.* 2006, Pearrow and Pollack 2009, Dworkski-Riggs and Langhout 2010, Langhout and Thomas 2010, Mallan, Singh and Giardina 2010, Guta, Flicker and Roche 2013), these approaches are positively considered to provide possibilities for young people's empowerment through developing their influence over the types of health services they use, with a particular emphasis on promoting partnerships with teachers, health professionals and other adults.

Participatory and more collective approaches to empowerment, however, reveal a number of complications for understanding the concept's relationship to young people's health. First, such approaches uncritically assume that young people want to be and indeed will be empowered through the process of defining and controlling their own agendas. Not only does this suggest that all young people want to be involved in shaping health-related agendas – an assumption that has not been empirically investigated – but this approach further assumes that young people will always know what they want (and what is best for health) and that through this process they will make 'healthy choices'.

Second, processes of CCR and agenda setting are often based on the facilitation of partnership working to achieve collective goals (Laverack 2009, Wiggins 2011). This approach not only denies the problematic nature of much partnership working and the power of professionals to assert their perspectives in such processes (see for example Ashworth, Longmate and Morrison 1992, Gregory 2000, Pease 2002, Laverack 2009) but also assumes that common goals can be identified and addressed.

Recent evidence highlights a disjunction between young people's concerns and those of policymakers, health professionals and other adults working with young people, such as teachers (Aynsley-Green *et al.* 2000, Kirby *et al.* 2003, Chawla *et al.* 2005, Sixsmith *et al.* 2007, Wills *et al.* 2008). In the United Kingdom, work by Percy-Smith (2006, 2007), for example, indicates that young people's health-related concerns draw attention to issues of stress, bullying and negative stereotypes of young people, whereas professionals more readily identify government-led priority areas such as drugs, alcohol, smoking and sex as being most pertinent to young people's health and lives.

This disjunction may inadvertently place professionals in an ambiguous position, with potentially contradictory accountabilities in attempting to meet political priorities whilst simultaneously trying to address the different (and potentially opposing) concerns and priorities identified by young people themselves. Cavet and Sloper (2004), for example, pointed to a number of ways in which young people's concerns have been marginalized in the development of local health services in England, including the failure of decision-makers to listen to young people and take their concerns seriously – a finding widely supported elsewhere in the literature (see Alderson 2000, Kirby *et al.* 2003, Boylan and Ing 2005, Chawla *et al.* 2005). Consequently, young people's experiences of participation often amount to little more than concessionary acts and tokenism (see Hart 1997) because political priorities and targets often take precedence.

It therefore seems somewhat problematic that those in a position to facilitate the necessary prerequisites for empowerment, such as health professionals and educators, may also work (deliberately or otherwise) to undermine any such empowerment. Professionals working with young people may in fact be representative of the very sources of power some young people may wish to challenge (Pinkey 2011). For instance, Boylan and Ing (2005) found that young people's main concerns often rest upon the unwillingness of adults to listen to their points of view and to take their perspectives seriously rather than any concerns about services per se (see also Cavet and Sloper 2004, Pinkey 2011).

Evidence of this kind highlights a further set of prerequisites for empowerment based on a *power over* conceptualization. Arguably, in order to demonstrate possibilities for empowerment, professionals working with young people need to be in a position to modify and change predefined policy concerns in accordance with young people's perspectives on health. This necessitates professionals working with young people to listen to and provide young people with the necessary access to information, knowledge and services to define and act on their concerns. This knowledge must be readily and effectively communicated but often has been found to be lacking based on dominant assumptions about young people's abilities to understand 'complex' information (Curtis *et al.* 2004, Hine, Lemetti and Trikha 2004).

Furthermore, any information and knowledge conveyed to young people may be selective, ultimately reflecting dominant assumptions about young people that typically construct them as being wilful, irrational and ignorant – and further positions them as either risky or at risk (Kelly 2000, 2003, 2006). In England, Curtis *et al.* (2004) found that health professionals are often partial in the information presented to young people in order to 'protect' them from having to make 'adult' decisions. Consequently, by highlighting available choices and providing 'appropriate' health-related knowledge, professionals may (consciously or unconsciously) determine young people's choices. This serves to question whether notions of empowerment based on processes of CCR can be anything but expert-led.

A fourth and final point concerning participatory and collective approaches to empowerment based on notions of CCR is the tendency to homogenize young people, thereby ignoring important differences that may exist between young people of different cultural and social backgrounds. Through the emphasis on bringing together 'disempowered' groups, CCR requires young people themselves to unite as a collective in order to identify the commonality of their marginalized position. Not only does more recent evidence drawing on poststructuralist perspectives suggest this would be a significant challenge as young people display a number of individual identities (Bauman 1996, Abbott-Chapman, Denholm and Wyld 2008) and occupy multiple subjective positions (Baxter 2002, Currie, Kelly and Pomerantz 2011), but (rather ironically) these collective notions of empowerment appear to necessitate young people's alignment with a position of 'powerlessness'. This, theoretically at least, may inhibit the initiation of empowerment by young people themselves who may not wish to see or define themselves as being powerless. It therefore seems that any notion of empowerment based on processes of CCR and *power over* perspectives may inadvertently support the idea that young people lack power, which, rather paradoxically, is the very position such a process seeks to challenge.

Power against or power through? Young people's resistance as empowerment

A final and now growing area of literature on empowerment, young people and health examines young people's varying forms of resistance to dominant relations of power – pointing to some possibilities for empowerment based on a *power through* conceptualization as young people (re)define, negotiate and resist power relations within the context of their everyday lives (see Ungar and Teram 2000, Allen 2003a and b, 2007, Renold 2004, Youdell 2005, Jackson 2006, Doull and Sethna 2011).

Moments of resistance, a concept extensively discussed in the youth literatures (Hall and Jefferson 1976, Aggleton and Whitty 1985, Aggleton 1987, Scott 1990, Raby 2002, 2005), illustrate active challenges to the imposition of power and control over young people. In relation to health, examples of young people's resistance to official health promotion messages can be seen in their accounts of their health-related practices. Katainen (2006), for example, highlighted how young people's accounts of smoking represent a mark of 'true' autonomy as young people critically question, and indeed resist, official health discourses through continuing to smoke. Similarly, in relation to alcohol, research from Sweden exemplifies how young people's accounts of their drinking behaviours reflect their abilities to negotiate and redefine health risks in accordance with normalized patterns of behaviour in the context of their everyday lives (Bogren 2006). Other research from Canada and England highlights the importance young people attach to their social positioning and how, through engaging in particular health practices, young people can negotiate and adopt more powerful social positions (Room and Sato 2002, Haines *et al.* 2009, Stead *et al.* 2011).

These examples of young people's forms of resistance to dominant health discourses may point to some possibilities for empowerment, but also illustrate how health promotion may perversely exacerbate the very behaviours it seeks to address (Crossley 2001b, 2002, Thompson and Kumar 2011). Crossley (2002, p. 1482) argued that didactical health promotion messages inevitably spur people's desire for rebellion as a marker of their independence and autonomy. Evidence of this kind thus creates two further difficulties for understanding possibilities for empowerment based on a *power through* conceptualization.

First, although young people's resistance to health promotion may well be seen as a logical response to the authority and control imposed on their lives, this resistance may ultimately serve to work against the promotion of health according to official perspectives (such as not smoking, drinking moderately, unsafe sex), thereby questioning the assertion that empowerment results in positive health outcomes in line with official discourses.

Second, empirical work drawing upon Foucault's (1991) notions of 'truth regimes' highlights how young people's resistance may be readily dismissed by dominant protectionist discourses as an indication of young people's lack of knowledge and rationality to act as autonomous, responsible beings (Lee 2001, Raby 2002, 2005). Consequently, young people's rejection of official health advice may present a significant barrier to empowerment (based on a *power through* conception) because their challenges may be readily accepted as evidence of their lack of knowledge, maturity and ability to determine their own health-related concerns. Paradoxically, young people's resistance to health promotion, although indicating possibilities for empowerment, may inadvertently support the dominant assertion that they are in fact 'at risk', thereby strengthening the dominant discourse about young people and health that any empowerment may seek to challenge.

Identifying young people's own understandings of health and priorities for health promotion may remain problematic when offering different perspectives to those articulated in dominant health discourses – a crucial concern further interrogated in subsequent chapters. Consequently, as Currie, Kelly and Pomerantz (2011) indicated, young people's attempts to push against boundaries of acceptable behaviours does not necessarily mean that dominant power regimes have been challenged, let alone transformed (p. 303).

Conclusion

This chapter has charted some of the major contributions to the theorization of power in order to help advance the conceptualization of empowerment. The analysis thus far has drawn on a tripartite perspective of power (*power to, power over, power through*) informed by Steven Lukes's (2005) radical view of power. This framework of power is considered especially appropriate for capturing and synthesizing different forms of power and provides the conceptual frame for further interrogating empowerment's relationship to young people's health in Part Two of the book.

Informed by this tripartite perspective of power, in this chapter I have further sought to examine more critically the existing empirical literature on empowerment and young people. By doing so, this form of analysis has uncovered a number of further theoretical tensions and operational challenges for understanding concepts of empowerment as they relate to young people's health and from differing conceptions of power. In particular, by engaging with a full-fledged theorization of power, the discussion has served to critically question the dynamics of empowerment and whether the concept has potential to promote young people's health – highlighting too how young people's possible challenges to dominant forms of power may unwittingly support, rather than transform, dominant power relations.

These emergent tensions highlight the impetus for further theorization and empirical investigation to better unpack the possibilities for, and limitations of, empowerment and, crucially, to advance the understanding of the concept's relationship to, and relevance for, young people's health and health promotion.

Part II

Investigating power, empowerment and young people's health

Part Two of this book details an empirical investigation on empowerment, young people and health (Spencer 2011). Drawing on the theoretical base described in Part One, the chapters that follow describe the overall methodological approach to the enquiry, before analysing some of the key findings from the investigation. By analysing study findings, alongside Lukes's (2005) tripartite model of power, a new conceptual framework for understanding the concept of empowerment as it relates to young people's health is proposed (the focus of Chapter Eight). This new framework aims to address some of the thorny theoretical tensions identified in Part One of the book and crucially, to help better explain the relationship between empowerment and young people's health. The final chapter in this section considers the relevance of this new framework for health promotion more broadly.

4 The study

This chapter outlines the broad approach taken in an empirical enquiry that sought to unpack the arguments hitherto articulated in this volume. The goal of the investigation was to examine what might be the possibilities for, and limitations of, empowerment amongst young people from a tripartite perspective of power. In the discussion that follows, I share some important details about the study's underpinning epistemological approach and methodology, the research methods employed, sampling techniques and recruitment procedures, data collection and the methods of analysis. A thorough account of some of the ethical considerations relevant to this study is also given.

I commence with a short discussion of some of the key methodological concerns and the potential complexities of conducting research with young people as given in the existing research literature. Detailed reflection on some of the complexities encountered in this particular study, including consideration of some of the likely limits to the study, are given in the book's concluding chapter (Chapter Nine).

Researching young people's health and empowerment

In recent years, much has been written on conducting research with young people (Lewis and Lindsay 2000, Fraser *et al.* 2004, Soto and Swadener 2005, Christensen and James 2008). The increasing (political) emphasis on eliciting children's and young people's 'voices' on topical concerns (see for example Department of Health [DH] 2004a, 2010b, Australian Government 2010) has triggered a proliferation of research conducted *with*, rather than *on*, young people. Often drawing on qualitative and participatory forms of enquiry, this now growing body of research has sought to enable children and young people to define the focus of much research on their everyday lives (see for example deWinter, Baerveldt and Kooistra 1999, Cree, Helen and Tisdall 2002, Punch 2002a and b, Chabot *et al.* 2012). Informed by perspectives from within the sociology of childhood (James and Prout 1997, Mayall 2002, Qvortrup, Cosaro and Honig 2009), this body of research typically positions young people as being active agents within the research process and often emphasizes the value of interpretive methods of enquiry for eliciting young people's perspectives (Mayall 1994, 1996, France, Bendelow and Williams 2000, Morrow 2001, Barker and Weller 2003, Alderson 2008, Christensen and James 2008).

Despite many of these underpinning participatory principles, this area of literature also points to a number of challenges when seeking to engage children and young people in research. Difficulties in establishing access and recruiting young people, coupled with barriers imposed by 'gate-keepers' such as parents and teachers, for example, demonstrate how young people's participation in research can be heavily constrained by external factors, including the decision often made by adults about whether young people's participation in research is deemed 'appropriate' (see Masson 2000, Smith, Monaghan and Broad 2003, Duncan *et al.* 2009, McCarry 2012).

Likewise, the complexities of gaining informed consent and asymmetries of power between an adult researcher and younger participant are frequently highlighted in the literature for their potential threats to reliability and validity (Barker and Weller 2003, Robinson and Kellett 2004, Flewitt 2005, Harcourt and Conroy 2005, Alderson and Morrow 2011, Watts 2011, McCarry 2012). Although increasing attention is accorded to ascertaining young people's perspectives, this emic[1] approach can be problematic as a consequence of such power differentials (see Harden *et al.* 2000, Balen *et al.* 2006, Sixsmith *et al.* 2007, Dentith, Measor and O'Malley 2009). The potential effects of power arising from, amongst other things, an adult researcher eliciting perspectives from younger participants are thus now part of the well-documented concerns about conducting research with young people (Soto and Swadener 2005, Dentith, Measor and O'Malley 2009).

The study

Against this background, the present study's concern for empowerment, young people and health sought to elicit young people's own understandings of health and enquire into how such meanings may be shaped and defined within the context of young people's everyday lives. The underpinning interpretive epistemology and abductive research strategy (Blaikie 2007) therefore took young people's own ways of seeing and knowing as its starting point for understanding concepts of health and empowerment.

Broadly defined, interpretivism advocates the importance of understanding the subjective meanings behind social action and concerns itself with the description and interpretation of human behaviour and action. A central tenet of this epistemology is that human action is meaningful and that individuals act on, and in relation to, meanings given to social action (Ezzy 2002). From this perspective, meanings given to social phenomena are not considered to be fixed and/or absolute truths but are continuously shaped and reshaped within the process of interaction and within different social contexts (Ezzy 2002, Duncan 2007).

By taking young people's own understandings and meanings of health as the starting point, the study's abductive research strategy further sought to align with many of the original theoretical underpinnings of empowerment (Gomm 1993, Labonte 1989, 1993, Laverack 2004, 2007). However, drawing on Schütz's (1963a and b) first and second order constructs (see also Weber 1947, Rex 1971, Giddens 1976a and b), this abductive logic further requires a hermeneutic dialogue to occur between lay concepts and meanings (first order concepts) and technical concepts and interpretations (second order concepts); (Blaikie 2007, p. 101). As Rex (1971, 1974) has argued, although social theories should be based on the everyday meanings of individuals, these in themselves may be influenced and determined by wider social structures and relations of power. An abductive logic therefore acknowledges the potential limits of people's understanding of their social world and points to the need for researchers to be critical of lay accounts. Consequently, respondents' accounts may be considered partial because of various forms of *power* that may play out in them.

The school setting

The proliferation of school-based research in recent times (see Testa and Coleman 2006, Austen 2009, Milstein 2010) has highlighted the school environment as an important context in which to investigate young people's health. Specifically, the centrality of schools in young people's everyday lives (Pearrow and Pollack 2009), their importance as contexts for the development of young people's health-related knowledge and practices (Hagquist and Starrin 1997, Maes and Lievens 2003, Allen 2007, Rowling 2009), and the recent focus on schools as health promotion settings, particularly in the UK context (Aggleton *et al.* 1998, 2000, Department for Education and Skills/Department of Health [DfES/DH] 2005, Warwick *et al.* 2005) suggested the relevance of the school setting as being one important research context in which to undertake the study.

One large secondary school with a diverse socioeconomic attachment area provided the initial context for the study. The school was situated in a market town in central England with a population of approximately 46,235 (Office for National Statistics [ONS] 2011). The town itself is surrounded by a number of affluent rural communities, masking the level of deprivation in the area – with two of the six wards in the town being ranked within the 20% most deprived areas in the country (*ibid.*). The town is well supported by major transport links, attracting a number of large-scale industries, so unemployment rates in the town are lower than the UK national average.

The school caters to this diverse local population and has approximately 1,248 students on roll (53.0% male, 47.0% female), of whom 261 attend the school's on-site sixth form centre[2] (Department for Education [DfE] 2013). The school is the largest of three secondary schools in the town. The majority of students live within one of the town's six wards, with some students travelling by bus from the surrounding (more affluent) villages. The percentage of students from minority ethnic backgrounds is higher than most schools in the local authority area, as is the number of students with special educational needs. The proportion of students eligible for free school meals reflects the national average. In 2012, 49.0% of students achieved five or more GCSEs[3] grades A Star (A*) to C, including English and Maths (which was lower than the English national average of 58.8% [DfE 2013]). The school was rated as 'satisfactory' in its most recent Ofsted report[4] and was granted Healthy Schools Status[5] in 2006.

Access into the school was achieved through contact with the school's vice principal. A series of meetings involving the vice principal, the school's director of learning, the pastoral manager, and the Child Protection and Welfare officer were arranged and took place prior to fieldwork. During these meetings, the study's purpose and arrangements for recruitment and informing potential participants and their parents or guardians were discussed and agreed.

Despite the advantages of recruiting from a school setting, it was important to acknowledge that research carried out in such a context carries particular (methodological) challenges. In particular, research undertaken in school contexts can unknowingly mirror dominant discourses that privilege adult authority (Allen 2007, 2008, Jupp 2007, Milstein 2010). Indeed, the school environment may be one where young people have relatively little control (Darbyshire, MacDougall and Schiller 2005) and therefore feel pressured to participate in research or to give 'correct' answers (David, Edwards and Alldred 2001).

Of particular importance to this study was the potential for responses given by school-based participants to be influenced by dominant 'healthy schools' rhetoric and the related risk-reduction discourses found in many schools in the United Kingdom (see DfES/DH, 2005). Furthermore, a prime focus on the school environment arguably downplays the potential significance of other, less formal, contexts in which young people's health may be shaped and experienced (Curtis and Jones 1998). In light of these concerns, fieldwork also took place in a number of surrounding community settings. These alternative contexts included popular social settings for young people such as local parks, the town centre, roller disco and sports and youth clubs. In addition, a number of social events such as music and dance concerts, birthday parties and the school prom provided key sites for fieldwork.

The participants

A purposive sampling frame enabled the development of a theoretically informed sample based on the following criteria – age, gender and social position.

Age

The sampling strategy aimed to recruit young people between the ages of 15 and 16 years (the last year of compulsory schooling in the United Kingdom). This age group was identified as being most appropriate for exploring the study's aim for two key reasons. First, as I described in Chapter Two, this age group has been the focus of much recent health promotion activity, with a specific focus on empowerment and reducing young people's engagement with risky health behaviours (see DH 2004a, DfES/DH 2005). Second, in the UK, young people in this age group are statutorily defined as 'nonadult' by virtue of their age alone (i.e., because they are under the age of 18 years). Drawing on contributions from the sociology of childhood (Alanen and Mayall 2001, Mayall 2002, Qvortrup, Cosaro and Honig 2009), this socially constructed nonadult status was deemed especially important to the study's main theoretical concern with concepts of empowerment and, in particular, the examination of how power relations between young people and adults might shape the possibilities for, and limitations of, empowerment amongst young people.

Gender

Both young men and women were recruited to the study for three key reasons. First, gender is widely considered to be an important determinant of health practices, perspectives and outcomes (Pascoe 2007, Charles and Walters 2008, Alexander *et al.* 2010, Knight *et al.* 2012, deVisser and McDonnell 2013, Oliffe *et al.* 2013), and the significance of gendered power relations in young people's experiences of health (in)equities has been well documented (Tolman 1999, Amos and Bostock 2007, Doull 2009, Landstedt, Asplund and Gådin 2009). Second, the literature points to some important differences between the perspectives of boys and girls on health and their health-related practices (Dixey *et al.* 2001, Rugkåsa *et al.* 2003, Shearer *et al.* 2005, Nichter *et al.* 2006). Third, in much of the literature to date, empowerment has been the focus of much work with either young men *or* most often young women[6] (see Hyde *et al.* 2005, Currie, Kelly, and Pomerantz 2006). Based on a fixed-sum model of power, the examination of either young men or young women's empowerment excludes the exploration of the ways in which gender may offer potentially opposing (or even synergistic) possibilities for empowerment for boys *and* girls.

Social position

To date, much has been written about the potential significance of young people's (lack of) self-esteem and confidence in relation to the possibilities for empowerment and influencing their engagement with practices deemed risky to their health (Wild *et al.* 2004, Jayakody *et al.* 2005). As I have argued elsewhere, this area of research has a tendency to downplay the more social meanings young people attach to their health-related practices (see Shoveller *et al.* 2004, 2010, Ingham 2006, Marston, King and Ingham 2006, Austen 2009, Stead *et al.* 2011, Nelson, MacDonald and Abbott 2012), including the possibility that young people may be demonstrating high self-esteem if they choose to engage in practices deemed risky or harmful to health (see McGee and Williams 2000, Turner and Gordon 2004). The widespread attention given to (developing) young people's self-esteem and confidence therefore fails to acknowledge how these inherently individualized concepts can be understood as emanating from profoundly social aspects linked to young people's social position in any given context (see Shoveller *et al.* 2004) and how, in turn, this social positioning may shape the subsequent possibilities for, and limitations of, their empowerment.

The sampling strategy therefore sought to recruit and compare the perspectives and experiences of young people from different social positions within the school context. One way of recruiting young people occupying different positions within this setting was to use the school's own cohort system. In this school, students were assigned to two main cohorts, which were further subdivided into three distinct pathways, hereafter referred to as Gold, Silver and Bronze groups (see Table 1 for a description of these groups and composition of group discussions). This cohort system was distinct from other (academic) streaming processes in place at the school that further positioned students according to their academic abilities (i.e., 'top', 'middle' and 'bottom' sets). Students were placed within a cohort based on their academic and nonacademic achievements (this included awards for sports, dance, drama and music) and their participation in extra-curricular activities. This positioning within the school system determined students' timetables and thus peer groupings and friendships. Potential participants were drawn from these three pathways as described in Table 1.

Professional sample

An interdisciplinary group of professionals working with, and for, young people's health in the school's locality were also recruited into the study (*n* = 18). Professionals working with young people are often considered to be well placed to comment on young people's health circumstances (Sixsmith *et al.* 2007). However, some recent research has revealed how young people's perspectives on health may differ considerably from those of adults working with young people (see Percy-Smith 2006, 2007, Wills *et al.* 2008).

Professional perspectives were elicited from the following individuals: school teachers, teaching assistants, school learning mentor, school counsellors, the school's pastoral manager, welfare officer, medical officer, members of the school management team, the head of Personal, Health and Social Education (PHSE), head of Student Support Services, the Social and Emotional Aspects of Learning (SEAL) coordinator, local youth workers, detached youth drug and alcohol specialists and the local authority county

Table 1 Study Groups and Composition of Group Discussions

Gold Group	Silver Group	Bronze Group[1]
(Refers to the 'top' students as demonstrated by their academic and non-academic achievements and participation in extra-curricular activities).	*(Refers to students considered to be less academic and who do not readily participate in extra-curricular activities).*	*(Refers to those students considered marginalized from school and unlikely to achieve academic qualifications and often disengage from school life as a consequence).*
Boys (*n* = 7)	Boys (*n* = 7)	Boys (*n* = 7)
Girls (*n* = 7)	Girls (*n* = 6)	Girls (*n* = 5)
Mixed (4 girls, 4 boys)	Mixed (4 girls, 4 boys)	Nil
Total *n* = 22	Total *n* = 21	Total *n* = 12

First published by Emerald Publishing Limited.

1 The Bronze group constituted a smaller number of students compared with the relative numbers of students in both the Gold and Silver groups. All students in the Bronze group regularly attending school (i.e., at least 1 day a week) took part in focus group discussions (*n* = 12). A mixed focus group discussion with both boys and girls was not conducted because of the smaller number of students in this group and as a consequence of a stated preference by the girls in this group to be interviewed separately from the boys.

councillor for young people. Individual interviews were conducted at the respective place of work of each professional. The key purpose and focus of these interviews was to ascertain the perspectives of adults working with young people on issues linked to health and to compare their consistency of match with those of younger participants.

The methods

The aims of the study were addressed using a number of close-focused, ethnographic methods, including focus group discussions, individual interviews and observational techniques. The decision to use such methods was guided by the interpretive approach to the enquiry in addition to the now growing body of literature on research with young people which points to the value of these methods for sensitively and effectively ascertaining young people's perspectives (Greene and Hogan 2005, Alderson 2008, Christensen and James 2008). Here, I provide a short description of these methods to highlight some of the relative strengths of these techniques before detailing how these methods were employed during fieldwork.

Focus groups

Focus groups emphasize the exploration of shared meanings and group in-teraction within the data collection process and typically involve a group of participants (usually six to eight) being asked about their perspectives, beliefs and attitudes on a defined topic of interest (Krueger and Casey 2009, Bryman 2012, Cresswell 2012). The strength of the focus group method lies in its ability to examine processes of group interaction and the ways in which participants' responses are expressed in relation to the perspectives of other group members (Hyde *et al.* 2005). If well facilitated, focus groups offer the possibility for participants to agree, modify or challenge the views expressed by others, thereby enabling the elicitation of a range of different perspectives on the topic of interest (Bloor *et al.* 2004).

In relation to eliciting perspectives on health issues, there has been much support for the focus group method (see Kitzinger 1994, Crossley 2002, McLafferty 2004, Green and Thorogood 2009). The potential peer support available within a focus group compared with an individual interview is further highlighted in relation to research with young people and, specifically, for its potential to defuse power relations between an adult researcher and younger participants (Mayall 1994, 1996, Mauthner 1997, Armstrong, Hill and Secker 2000, David, Edwards and Alldred 2001, Hennessy and Heary 2005, Bagnoli and Clark 2010).

Despite the reported strengths of focus groups, it is important to consider some likely limitations of this method. A substantial research literature highlights concern about the effects of peers, dominant participants and group dynamics on the reliability and validity of qualitative data (Hammersley 1987, Sussman *et al.* 1991, Whittemore, Chase and Mandle 2001, Aguinaldo 2004, Bloor *et al.* 2004, Krueger and Casey 2009). The notion of 'group think' (Janis 1982), whereby collective responses may become more polarized than individual opinions, also raises serious concerns for validity. This has instigated much debate in the methodological literature concerning the use of either heterogeneous or more homogeneous groups (see Krueger and Casey 2009).

Individual interviews

In order to elicit more in-depth perspectives and, in part, to guard against possible limitations of group discussions, individual interviews were also conducted. The particular strength of the individual interview lies in its potential for detailed exploration of personal perspectives in a manner less susceptible to the peer influence potentially present within focus groups (Bryman 2012). Conducting individual interviews was therefore deemed important for minimizing any potential group effects and likewise, individual interviews have been used extensively in health-related research with young people (Wright, O'Flynn and MacDonald 2006, Johansson, Brunnberg and Eriksson 2007). Further, individual interviews were considered important for discussion of topics potentially too inhibiting to talk about in a group context.

Again a note of caution is offered with respect to this method. Some evidence suggests that participants in individual interviews may be tempted to present and conform to official perspectives (Harden *et al.* 2000). This again raises concerns for validity as accounts given may merely reiterate what participants think the researcher wishes to hear. Although individual interviews are less subject to group effects, the researcher's presence may in itself have an important influence on the responses elicited. Indeed, it is arguably more difficult for participants (and even the researcher) to challenge the views expressed or diverge from the particular line of questioning within the context of an individual interview (Bryman 2012). This form of reactivity has been raised as a particular concern in research with young people, where responses given in individual interviews have been found to be more inhibited (see for example Armstrong, Hill and Secker 2000, Harden *et al.* 2000, Westcott and Littleton 2005).

Observation

Although I acknowledge the possible limitations of group and individual interviews, such methods offer the potential for a more in-depth exploration of young people's perspectives on health and empowerment. However, because the narratives elicited from young people in these contexts might themselves be influenced to some extent by the processes of power the study sought to explore, observational methods were also integrated into the study.

Methods of observation are increasingly utilized as a key component of qualitative research (Colic-Peisker 2004, Walford 2007, 2008, Milstein 2010). Originating in the field of social anthropology, observation methods are often used for investigating particular social groups and contexts (Agar 1996, Hammersley 2006). More recently, observational methods have been employed successfully to explore concepts of health, risk and empowerment amongst young people in varying social contexts (see Clatts and Sotheran 2000, Hodkinson 2005, Ashcraft 2006, Groes-Green 2009, 2012, Briggs 2010, Woodgate and Leach 2010, Watts 2011, Bennett and Gough 2013).

The methodological literature distinguishes between various forms of observation with different degrees of participation and structure (see Angrosino 2007, Gillham 2008). Nonparticipant observation involves a degree of distancing of the researcher as he or she acts as an 'onlooker' of events. In contrast, participant observation acknowledges the presence of the researcher as he or she actively engages with participants in the immediate context. Participant observation does not assume that the researcher is simply assimilated into the context or becomes a member of the group under investigation,[7] but this approach importantly acknowledges the contribution of and potential reactivity caused by the researcher.

Periods of observation further necessitate the development of trusting relationships with participants, including a process of role negotiation and acceptance of the researcher as a 'legitimate peripheral participant' (Dhand 2007, p. 1; see also Duncombe and Jessop 2012). The researcher's 'deep involvement' stemming from observational techniques has been the subject of much criticism of this method, particularly from positivist traditions that highlight the subjectivity of such involvement (Brewer 2005). However, as Tucker (2007) and others (see Walkerdine, Lucey and Melody 2002, Blackman 2007, Denzin 2007, Holland 2007, Altheide and Johnson 2013) have noted, the researcher's subjectivity is seen to be an inevitable and epistemologically significant part of the research process, and its effects can be guarded against through the researcher's analytical distance and reflexivity – a point to which I return and reflect on in this book's closing chapter.

Fieldwork

A pilot study was conducted to assess the relative strengths (and identify limitations) of the proposed research design. Fieldwork took place over a period of 6 months. Initially, a series of eight focus groups were conducted with 55 young people (see Table 1). These focus group discussions served to familiarize participants to the research and researcher in addition to identifying key areas to be followed through and interrogated in individual interviews. Efforts were made, through observation work and consultation with the school's vice principal, to ensure group interviews comprised participants well known to each other but who did not constitute close friendship groups. This strategy was used to help guard against the effects of 'group think' on data validity (Janis 1982). Field notes were made to examine potential concerns for data validity and detailed thoughts about any extraneous factors pertaining to researcher and participant interaction, group dynamics and interaction, expression and the intensity of responses.

Following focus group discussions, participants were invited to take part in individual interviews. These individual interviews enabled more detailed exploration of issues raised during group discussions in addition to identifying further issues considered potentially too inhibiting to discuss in a group context. All participants involved in focus group discussions agreed to participate in a subsequent individual interview ($n = 55$).

Focus groups and individual interviews took place in a quiet meeting room in the school. Additional discussions also took place with participants during periods of observation. A short summary of each discussion was given and verified at the end of each session to ensure that the main points discussed had been acknowledged in the context of participants' accounts. This was achieved through noting participants' responses during interviews and then providing a verbal summary of these notes at the end of discussions for clarification with participants. At times, this enabled participants to further explain their meanings in relation to areas discussed – serving to extend and deepen the responses elicited. Teachers were not present during these discussions because their presence might have affected discussions and responses.

All focus group and interview discussions were audio-recorded (with consent of participants) and transcribed verbatim soon after the session wherever possible. This prompt transcription enhanced the quality and re-liability of transcriptions because immediate recall of the discussion was more readily available and was supported by the field notes. These strate-gies aimed to minimize any potential 'losses' to data collected through, for example, any inaudible recordings. The timely transcription also enabled identification of any emerging themes or discussion areas to further pursue during the time of fieldwork, in addition to clarifying any inconsistencies and ambiguities in participants' responses that might have limited the qual-ity of the subsequent analysis. This technique, amongst others, confirmed the consistency of match between my own interpretations and participants' meanings – often referred to as 'member checking' in the literature (Denzin and Lincoln 2011).

A literature review on recent research on empowerment, young people and health guided the development of interview and focus group discus-sion guides. Questions explored were piloted with a small group of young people from the same geographical area as the main sample but who were not involved in the main study. In order to remain faithful to the exploratory nature of the enquiry and to minimize my own potential influence on re-sponses, the interview guides remained fairly unstructured (Robson 2011).

As described in Chapter One, this study positioned young people's own frames of reference as central to understanding the concept of empower-ment as it relates to health. Drawing on more positive conceptualizations of health, such as those provided by Antonovsky (1979) and Seedhouse (2001), the interview guide sought to capture the potentially multiple mean-ings young people attach to the broad concept of health, including both positive and negative dimensions. Specifically, the approach to the study sought to decentralize dominant understandings of health as 'the absence of disease' by tapping into young people's perspectives on the more affective aspects of health – including their thoughts on being well and not feeling well. These affective states of health have been highlighted as being impor-tant, not just for supporting physical health but also for their role in shaping health-related practices (Kubzansky and Kawachi 2000, Salovey *et al.* 2000, Richman *et al.* 2005). The study therefore sought to capture the totality of health as seen by young people – be that ill health or feeling or being well. In addition, given that the concept of empowerment seeks to start from people's own concerns (Labonte 1989, 1994, Laverack 2009), this approach to questioning was further considered to be more in line with the original underpinning principles of empowerment.

In light of these noted concerns, and in order to minimize response bias and avoid priming around official or dominant notions of health, respon-dents were asked to discuss their own understandings of 'feeling and being well' and 'feeling good' in addition to their understandings of 'not being or feeling well' or 'feeling not their normal self'. This included identifying factors that participants perceived to influence, promote or constrain their feelings of being well. A similar approach had been successfully used in earlier research by Aggleton *et al.* (1996) and Spencer (2008) in explorations of young people's perspectives on health (see also Cameron, Mathers and Parry 2008). Participants were further asked about opportunities to influence matters of importance to them both at home and school and in the community more generally. Participants' suggestions for parents, teachers or the government in relation to promoting young people's health were also elicited during discussions.

Observation of young people's interactions with their peers and teachers were carried out over the course of the whole school day. This involved observing and interacting with students as they came into school, during registration and lesson time as well as breaks and lunchtimes; this sometimes involved observations away from school grounds. Observational work often continued immediately after school as I was increasingly invited by participants to accompany them into the town centre and before they went home. At times, observation work involved a degree of participation. For instance, during fieldwork in out-of-school contexts, participants often invited me to play table tennis or cricket or go roller-skating, amongst other activities. Observations focused on young people's everyday encounters and interactions with others – both adults and peers. This included observing the reactions of teachers, peers and others to young people as they went about their daily lives.

Observations were carefully documented as far as was feasible at that time. Within the school context, notes were taken during lessons relating to young people's interactions with peers and adults, in addition to any forms of reactivity arising from my own presence in the school setting. In out-of-school contexts, such as local parks or parties, notes were made using a mobile phone whereby observations and discussions of young people's interactions and practices were entered into the phone. Using a mobile phone offered a less intrusive and more socially acceptable technique to document observations in real time. A detailed summary and reflection was written at the end of each day to capture key thoughts in relation to the theoretical and methodological concerns of the study. This included a reflection on my own position in the field to consider the ways in this positioning might have affected the responses elicited and observations made.

The purpose of these observations was to further understand the various ways processes of power operated and impacted upon participants' perspectives, beliefs and practices. These observations may say something about the importance of context (and young people's position within that context) to the possibilities for, and limitations of, empowerment. For instance, examples of young people's opportunities to influence events or subvert the normal order of the social context, along with young people's challenges, acceptance or compliance with various rules and authority operating in any given context, were also noted.

Observation enabled me to talk to young people in a more 'naturalistic' way (Gillham 2008) and provided some safeguard against the documented limitations of the more 'formal' context of interviews (see Harden *et al.* 2000). Importantly, discussions with participants during observation periods enabled me to access young people's thoughts and views on events occurring in real time. This provided a more detailed and authentic account of young people's perspectives, in contrast to solely relying on recall and reporting of events during the context of an interview.

Methods of analysis

A short summary of each discussion was prepared following each session to capture the main themes (Krueger and Casey 2009). Discussions were transcribed verbatim immediately after the sessions wherever possible. Transcriptions were then checked against the recording for accuracy and amended as necessary. In line with an abductive research strategy, data were analysed using a multistage process. Drawing on participants' perspectives, the first stage involved a descriptive analysis whereby patterns and connections were identified from the data itself. This first stage of analysis served to summarize the data and highlight emerging themes (Grbich 2012). For example, initial readings of transcripts highlighted a number of broad topic areas, including the police, school, friends, parents, smoking, alcohol and having fun.

Second, a thematic analysis was undertaken whereby responses given in focus group and individual interviews were coded (Holliday 2007). Next, emerging themes were categorized and organized according to the research questions. For example, themes from young people's discussions of feeling well included the topical categories of 'being happy' and 'having fun'. Similarly, young people's discussions of 'not feeling well' indicated the importance respondents attached to 'being judged'. These topical categories, and others, were further examined to highlight emerging subthemes (for example, *young and dumb, being bad*), which were then analysed for their implications for emic conceptualizations of health and empowerment. The third stage involved a theoretical analysis whereby emerging patterns and topical themes were examined drawing on Lukes's tripartite perspective of power (*power to, power over, power through*). Amongst other techniques, this stage of the analysis drew upon the review of the literature and policy texts to further reveal any similarities and inconsistencies between young people's accounts and current understandings of young people's health and empowerment.

A further comparative element of the analysis focused on the relationship between observations made and the accounts elicited within the school context and observations and accounts elicited from young people in out-of-school contexts. This involved coding and grouping data according to context to examine any emergent differences or consistencies across the data. The significance of gender and young people's social positioning as defined by their cohort grouping was also considered in light of the purposive sampling frame. This technique enabled a closer examination of any specific themes emerging from, for example, young men from a particular group with those of another group of young men, and similarly a comparison by gender.

The consistency of match between young people's perspectives and those offered by professionals was further compared. Accounts elicited from professionals were coded and categorized in line with the process described. First, emergent themes were compared against those elicited from young people. Second, professionals' accounts were analysed by drawing upon findings from a critical discourse analysis of health-related policy. This involved highlighting consistencies in data where accounts aligned with policy discourses as well as examining examples of any differences.

Ethical considerations

Ethical implications relevant to this study were considered in light of the now growing literature on research ethics relevant to research with children and young people (Christensen and Prout 2002, Hill 2005, Alderson and Morrow 2011, Watts 2011, Chabot *et al.* 2012). Ethical approval was sought and granted from a university faculty research ethics committee. The research was informed by the framework outlined by Alderson and Morrow (2011), which gives particular attention to ethics relevant to research with young people. A short account of these ethical considerations is given here to illuminate some of the potential challenges that may emerge during an investigation of this kind.

Informed consent

The notion of informed voluntary consent is central to the conduct of ethical research and demonstrates respect for an individual's right to self-determination and autonomy (Meyrick 2005). Gaining consent within a school environment can be problematic as the effects of active encouragement from teachers and/or peers may persuade or coerce an individual to participate (David, Edwards and Alldred 2001, France 2004, Meyrick 2005). In light of these documented concerns, written informed consent was obtained individually from participants prior to data collection. Furthermore, ascertaining written informed voluntary consent was not viewed as a single act of agreement on behalf of the participant but instead a process of continuous negotiation throughout the research period (Milstein 2010, Alderson and Morrow 2011).

In order to ensure consent was well informed, participants were provided with an information sheet outlining the purpose of the study and the nature of their involvement during class and assembly presentations. These class and assembly presentations served to inform all students and school staff about the research, even if they were not directly participating in the study.

These discussions drew specific attention to the implications of observational methods to ensure staff and students were aware at all times that the research was being carried out. Participants were given opportunities to ask questions prior to data collection sessions and were free to raise any points about the research at any time. It was made clear to all respondents that participation was voluntary and that they were free to withdraw from the study at any point and without giving reason. Particular attention was given to the processes of consent during observational work. As such, I consistently confirmed with participants that my presence (and purpose for my presence) was met with support by the young people involved in the study.

Written permission was obtained from the school prior to data collection. In addition, parents or guardians of potential participants were sent a letter and short description of the study and the nature of their son or daughter's involvement. Parents and guardians were provided with contact details and the opportunity to discuss the research in more detail during a parents' evening event held at the school. Potential participants were further encouraged to discuss their participation with their parents/guardians prior to giving their consent.

Confidentiality, privacy and anonymity

Conducting group-based research requires careful attention to issues of confidentiality, privacy and anonymity. Issues relating to confidentiality were therefore discussed in detail with participants prior to fieldwork. This discussion emphasized the importance of respecting all participants' opinions and nondisclosure of the content of the discussions outside of the group setting in order to preserve both individual and third-party confidentiality (Horowitz *et al.* 2003). In order to guard against the invasion of participants' privacy, during all observation periods I continuously checked with participants that my presence was welcomed and similarly reiterated that participants could at any point request for me to leave or cease observations. Anonymity was ensured through the omission of any identifying data, including participants' names and places from which data were collected. Data were stored in accordance with the requirements of the Data Protection Act (1998).

Protection from possible harm

The risk of distress, anxiety and embarrassment needs to be considered in all research, particularly when it involves young people (Alderson and Morrow 2011). Respondents were likewise informed prior to fieldwork that in the unlikely event of a participant becoming distressed or suffering possible harm, the participant could withdraw, and if necessary, the research would be interrupted. If such an event occurred, participants would be guided to the appropriate school or community support service as necessary. These points were again discussed in detail with participants prior to data collection sessions and further detailed on the study information sheets. During fieldwork, participants were also given an additional information sheet with contact details of a variety of local and national support services and helplines for young people should they wish to discuss any personal issues or concerns.

Participant and researcher safety

Observation in out-of-school contexts took place following a period of time spent with participants at school, which increased as the study progressed. This approach ensured participants were already familiar with the research before this part of the study was conducted. Prior to fieldwork, I acknowledged the possibility that during observational work (particularly in out-of-school settings) I might witness evidence of participants (and other young people) engaging in health-related practices deemed harmful, such as smoking or drinking alcohol. Interestingly, these concerns were not well supported by observations made during fieldwork, and (as subsequent chapters reveal) young people were often highly critical of the (adult) assumption that young people spend a significant amount of their time engaging in potentially risky health practices.

Potential risks to the safety of participants were, however, carefully considered before fieldwork. Because of this, observational work was largely carried out in public places, such as the town centre, or more organized social venues, such as the local roller-disco and sports and youth clubs. Other adults were often present in these contexts. Local police, community support workers and detached youth workers were informed of the research and were, at times, present during fieldwork.

Conclusion

This chapter has outlined the overall methodological approach to the enquiry, including a consideration of some of the now well-documented challenges of conducting research with young people. In particular, I have detailed some of the key decisions made in relation to issues of sampling and recruitment, methods of data collection and analysis. Fifty-five young participants took part in the study, sampled across three different groupings (Gold, Silver and Bronze) from within the school context. A number of alternative settings were also used as important fieldwork sites, including the local town centre, sports clubs and the roller-disco. In addition, professional perspectives were elicited from 18 adults working with young people in the study locality. I have further outlined some of the potential ethical issues the study may have raised. A more thorough account and reflection on some of the possible strengths and likely limitations of the approach described here are given in the book's concluding chapter.

5 Being happy and having fun

Young people's perspectives on health[1]

In this first of three chapters detailing study findings,[2] I focus specifically on young people's accounts of 'feeling well'. Three key arguments are made. First, by analysing young people's own understandings of health, some important prerequisites for empowerment are identified that on closer examination challenge current individualized conceptions or *power to* notions of the concept. Second, by stressing young people's own frames of reference when discussing health, we can begin to consider what might be young people's own (and potentially different) health-related concerns and priorities – indicating possibilities for empowerment based on a *power over* conceptualization. Third, these alternative perspectives on health highlight some counterhegemonic tendencies in young people's narratives and practices – pointing to some possibilities for collective forms of empowerment. Based on a *power through* conceptualization, these counterhegemonic tendencies are considered for their potential to shift and redefine (dominant) understandings of young people's health in line with their own perspectives.

Being happy

In this study, young people's accounts of feeling well were closely linked to the affective state of being happy. Specifically, being happy was largely understood by participants as 'feeling good about yourself'. Friendships and a sense of personal achievement were found to be of particular importance to these young people.

Researcher:	Can you tell me what feeling well means to you?
Wendy:	Being happy.
Sarah:	Yeah being happy.
Lucy:	Having lots of people around you that make you feel happy, so having like lots of friends and family.
Charlotte:	Having a laugh with them and being relaxed with them (Gold group).

Researcher: Can you tell me what feeling well means to you?
Lisa: Being happy, like just feeling well in yourself and achievement, if you've done something well . . . it makes you feel good about yourself (Gold group).

Young people's accounts of being happy suggested their everyday preference for more positive notions of health – typically framed in terms of developing a positive self-belief. Examining participants' interpretations of what they termed a 'belief in the self' highlighted three key ways in which young people sought to be happy: *knowing I can do something, looking good, and talking to others*. These three interpretations signalled some of the positive and more relational aspects of young people's health and specifically, their propensity to feel good in particular social situations.

Knowing I can do something

'Knowing I can do something' was frequently cited by young people as being a key aspect of being happy. In particular, doing well in sports and schoolwork pointed to some young people's involvement and achievements across a range of activities. Observations made in the school context revealed how many young people (particularly those in the Gold group) were often involved in music, dance and sporting events and frequently received commendations for their academic and nonacademic achievements.

Charlotte: Just knowing that I can believe in myself and that I can do something. 'Cos generally if I can do something that I'm quite confident in and I can go and do that as well as I can (Gold group).

Gina: If I know I'm doing bad in something and then I get a good grade in it, it gives me confidence, I think well I can do this (Gold group).

Doing well in schoolwork or sporting activities often resulted in praise and positive recognition from parents, teachers and friends. Here, young people's discussions of increases to their motivation and confidence to succeed seemed to be contingent upon the (positive) response and reinforcement by others, and not purely the attainment of a good grade.

Michael: In my speaking and listening that was the highest grade I ever got, and I just came in with a massive high, I was just glowing . . . then I started thinking about what my mum's and dad's gunna think and they're gunna give me a lot of praise. It's a chain reaction, you feel good, then you realize that they'll feel good, it makes you feel even better (Gold group).

David: I go home with a pack of commendations from the head of year, they say it's excellent. That's a sense of wow I've achieved something. I've made my parents proud (Silver group).

The relational aspects of developing a positive self-belief become clearer when contrasting the accounts and experiences of young people in the Gold group with those of the Bronze group. More often, young people in this latter group pointed to the lack of acknowledgment and limited opportunities for them to do well – frequently reporting that they rarely received positive comments from teachers and parent figures.

Kelly: Miss Gleeson [schoolteacher] saying about our confidence at school, what about us lot? Our confidence ain't right and they don't feel down for us.

Sonya: People call us the dumb half and that's why we call it the dumb half because our confidence ain't there (Bronze group).

Whilst these accounts may indicate some young people's uptake of those more individualized discourses surrounding self-confidence and self-esteem operating in the school context, these discussions also highlight the importance many young people attached to receiving positive recognition from adults. In these examples, developing and maintaining a positive self-belief appeared to be less a consequence of the individual doing well than the nature of the school environment, which (in this context at least) seemed to offer some young people greater opportunity to demonstrate their abilities to succeed. The reported lack of praise and recognition experienced by members of the Bronze group highlight the ways in which some young people's self-belief was closely linked to the (school) context in which any possibilities for empowerment may be realized.

Looking good

A second key element of young people's discussions of being happy tied to their concerns about their appearances. Young people in this study attached great importance to 'looking good' as a key element of their health (cf. Brooks and Magnusson 2007, Raby 2010). Some important differences were seen in the accounts given by boys from those given by the girls. These differences are examined separately here to indicate the ways in which young people's appearances were highly defined and regulated according to dominant gender norms.

For young women in this study, descriptions of looking good included following the latest styles of fashion, hair and make-up often depicted in popular celebrity magazines and the media more generally. Being perceived as attractive contributed to the girls' (social) positioning as these young women discussed how keeping up with the latest fashions not only enabled them to fit in with peers but also made them feel attractive to boys.

Lisa: I like it when you go out, getting all dressed up and doing my hair and make-up. It makes you feel good, you know if you think you look good and have nice clothes, and then you go out and meet people, you just feel more happy (Gold group).

Melissa: Like being able to go up to, for example, with boys and I was liking one of them, like if I look good, like to go over to them and just start chatting to them. . . . Like hair and make-up I think that's important for me because it makes you feel better if you're wearing hair extensions or make-up, it makes you feel good about yourself (Silver group).

These young women's frequent reference to dominant media images of attractive women, however, highlighted some contradictions in their narratives. On the one hand, media images of celebrities were discussed as creating 'pressure' and undermining their confidence, particularly when they felt their own appearance did not match up. However, these images were also described positively – offering possibilities for young women to develop their confidence by aligning their appearances with those of women depicted in the media. Whilst some girls reported that looking good was important for self-confidence, others seemed to suggest that an obsessive concern with looks revealed a lack of confidence in simply 'being yourself'. The particular value given to the appearances of attractive women in the media, however, restricted the acceptability of more individual forms of expression – which for other girls was seen as a 'true' mark of being happy with themselves. Consequently, some young women's displays of resistance to these dominant images (through the adoption of alternative styles – such as wearing loose-fitting jumpers, jeans and trainers along with the absence of any make-up or jewellery) were often met with criticism by others.

Melissa: If there's a certain fashion and someone's not wearing that fashion, then there can be a lot of bitchiness. . . . Like stuff people say, like if you's wearing some jeans that didn't fit you properly and people are like 'your jeans are a bit tight', it makes you feel bad, or when they say your hair makes you look pretty rough. Girls are really bitchy (Silver group).

For some girls who dressed differently, their alternative styles of dress seemed to leave them open to judgement, bitchiness and potential exclusion from peer groups. This reported bitchiness was often linked to girls' broader discussions of 'not feeling well' – pointing to some of the pressures experienced by these girls to look good as a mark of their popularity amongst peers. Consequently, the importance of aligning their appearances to one form of dominant femininity (largely based on attractive women in the media) seemed to create limits for young women's (individual) resistance to dominant gender norms – thus, limiting possibilities for individual expressions of empowerment. In contrast, possibilities for empowerment by conforming to, rather than resisting, these particular forms of femininity had the effect of reducing the social value of other young women's appearances. The resulting marginalization some girls experienced as a consequence of dressing differently ultimately had negative impacts on their reports of being happy – thereby raising some questions about whether such individual expressions of 'empowerment' have the potential to promote health in line with young people's own frames of reference.

These contradictory elements of young women's appearances indicated how some girls (particularly those in the Bronze group) appeared to have less opportunity to fit in with their peers as judgements about their appearances acted as an exclusionary device, denigrating them and their appearances as 'unattractive' and 'unpopular'.

Kelly:	They [Gold group] get all bought all their clothes; it's all about the styles they wear, the clothes. They judge people by what they look . . . and then when you get judged that's when it just lowers you down. It's like when you come to school people look at you and pick on you, you've got a different make of trainers, you've got a different make of clothes. Everyone's like, 'Why you wearing the cheap stuff?' and they're wearing the expensive stuff and then they judge you (Bronze group).

As Kelly's account indicates, for some young women the opportunity to align their appearances with these dominant images was closely tied to the affordability of preferred fashions, hairstyles and make-up. Young women in the Bronze group (and some girls in the Silver group), described having less (economic) opportunity to access and adopt these more expensive (gendered) appearances – often suggesting that other girls (such as those in the Gold group) could buy the types of clothes socially desired by all girls. As a consequence, the girls reported to feel and be excluded by other girls (and also excluded themselves) from particular social contexts on the grounds of having nothing to wear (cf. Archer, Hollingworth and Halsall 2007).

Researcher:	Can you say a bit more about the reaction from other girls?
Kirsten:	You feel less happy, you feel like you're worthless.
Hayley:	Because a lot of girls they are sort of classed, like downgraded.
Researcher:	What do you mean by downgraded?
Hayley:	Meaning they can't go out, like buy anything. They can't go out and buy the top brand make-up, they can't afford that, so it means you've got some girls who it's actually quite intimidating for those who can't have that (Silver group).

These reports of having nothing to wear were more closely linked to having nothing 'acceptable' to wear. Lack of money was not only seen to restrict opportunities to fit in with peer groups but also restricted engagement with social events because the girls believed they would be open to criticism based on their (unacceptable) appearances. Reported judgements made about the appearances of girls in the Bronze and Silver groups therefore appeared to 'fix' these young women into a more marginalized social position because their 'cheap' appearances (and assumed related identities) defined them as largely 'worthless' – with negative effects on their belief in themselves.

> *Carla:*   I don't like what people say about me, it's not very nice. I pretend it doesn't bother me when really it does, it makes me feel really bad (Bronze group).

For these girls, possibilities for empowerment were not only shaped in relation to their positioning amongst peers but were also influenced by financial means, which limited, and even denied, some girls' opportunities to negotiate valued (and potentially more empowered) social positions. The boundaries created by girls' (economic and gendered) appearances thus acted as a form of social exclusion and were used to draw (social) distinctions between different groups of girls. The social comparisons made about other young women's appearances indicated the way in which girls themselves, rather hypocritically, judged others by their appearances.

> *Kirsten:*   There is a lot of bitchiness. I try to avoid it but every girl bitches.
> *Researcher:*   And what are they doing when you say they're bitching?
> *Kirsten:*   If say you're friends with someone who isn't, she's not got much money and they like say 'Oh she's scruffy' and like 'Why you friends with her?'
> *Researcher:*   Can you say a bit more about that?
> *Kirsten:*   I've got a friend she has her own style, she doesn't follow the fashion and because of that they don't like me or my friend (Silver group).

This (self and peer) surveillance, whereby acceptable and unacceptable styles of dress were continuously scrutinized and regulated, was further heightened by attention from boys, which often brought about marked changes in some girls' appearance.

> At the end of the lesson Sonya gets changed. She tells me about Dean looking at her. She puts on a vest top and smiles at me; it seems quite obvious she is getting changed for Dean. As she leaves, she runs past me and says 'I don't care if he sees'. . . . During registration Sonya is smiling and seems excited. For the first time, she is wearing a skirt to school, has her hair down and is wearing make-up. (Field notes)

Here, changing their appearances appeared to enable some girls to affirm a more positive belief in the self, but in doing so, these potential expressions of 'empowerment' seemed to play into (and reproduce) dominant gender ideologies. Young women's role in the reproduction of these gender ideologies, however, was not always seen as negative because aligning with these highly gendered appearances enabled these girls to promote their health according to their own frames of reference (i.e., by feeling more attractive to their peers).

These gendered and class-based dimensions of young women's appearances illustrate some of the contradictory elements of young women's empowerment. Possibilities for young women's empowerment took place in contexts heavily defined by dominant gender norms, which placed many girls in contradictory and potentially vulnerable positions. The pressure stemming from the intense (self and peer) regulation of some girls' appearances appeared to hold profound implications for their positive beliefs in themselves and pointed to an important area in which challenges to young women's health were continuously negotiated and potentially threatened by the operation of dominant (economic and gendered) power relations.

In contrast to current theorizations of empowerment that describe the concept as a continuum moving from the individual to the collective (see Laverack 2009), these illustrations further highlight how individual and collective forms of empowerment can sometimes work against each other. In these examples, individual displays of young women's resistance to dominant norms concerning appearance (i.e., by wearing clothes that differed from those captured in popular media) set limits to any collective effort to challenge dominant understandings of femininity more broadly, as adopting these alternative appearances set them apart from their peers. In contrast, most young women's preference for adopting shared appearances that align with images of attractive women in the media (whilst indicating some possibilities for collective empowerment) also revealed the potential for this form of empowerment to reinforce, rather than challenge or transform, dominant gender norms.

Evidence of boys' concern with their appearance as an index of feeling well was also found in their accounts. In particular, young men's discussions of looking good highlighted the particular (social) value attached to various styles of dress, such as wearing a 'hoodie'[3] or 'flat peak'.[4] In their discussions of feeling well, young men also pointed to the significance of self and peer assessment of their appearances to the achievement of (positive) health.

Researcher: Can you tell me what feeling well means to you?
Nathan: If I'm looking good.
Researcher: And why's that important for you?

Nathan: If I don't look good, like if my hair's crap, I feel on a bit of a downer. Sometimes you can look rough and I don't want anyone to see me. That makes me feel bad. I can't go out looking like this (Silver group).

Young men's appearances similarly enabled them to negotiate valued social positions amongst peers. Consequently, when asked by teachers to remove items of nonschool uniform such as hooded sweatshirts, caps and flat peaks, some boys would object to such requests. Whilst peer assessment of their appearance was of central importance to these young men, teachers viewed the boys' resistance as an attempt to defy school rules and evidence of their 'disruptive' and 'unruly' behaviour. Consequently, in trying to maintain their appearances (which they linked directly to sustaining their own health), these young men unwittingly prompted a series of (negative) reactions by teachers and other adults.

Josh: It's just appearance, like first impression, that's basically *you*, then they're thinking oh he's gunna do this and do that (Bronze group).

Aaron: The only people I don't feel stereotyped by are people who look like me. I think it is something to do with the way you look (Bronze group).

As these accounts suggest, young men in this study often discussed times when they felt they had been judged negatively by virtue of wearing hoodies, tracksuits (*trackies*), and flat peaks. These young men's accounts illustrate how judgements made about their appearances reflected an important challenge to their health, with further implications for any related possibilities for empowerment.

Pete: It's like people they look at you and they just think 'pwoof' . . . They just judge you by the way you look.
Researcher: And what is it about the way you look?
Pete: Flat peak, trainers, trackies. Like a chav,[5] they just think you're one of those that stand round on corners, spitting at people, throwing things . . .
Researcher: Why do you think they think that about you?
Pete: Because they see us walking around with hoodies on, we're not bad people, we're good people, like don't judge a book by its cover (Silver group).

These reported judgements made about young men's appearances appeared to be closely linked to current public and political concern about young people's perceived involvement in antisocial and violent behaviour (see Messias *et al.* 2008 for example). This wider public concern about anti-social behaviour was, however, heavily criticized by these boys for support-ing the assumption that all young men are, or could be, violent criminals.

Dean: Because we're wearing hoodies, they class us and put us in a certain group that they would put criminals. They see us and think he's got a knife, is he gunna mug me, is he gunna stab someone 'cos he's wearing a hoodie (Bronze group).

Although following particular styles of dress (such as wearing the hoodie) enabled these boys to feel good about themselves and positively position themselves amongst peers, their accounts further indicated how wearing a hoodie left them open to criticisms from adults and the public more gener-ally. The tendency to problematize young men's appearances was further seen to impact on these boys' everyday lives because they frequently dis-cussed how these wider criticisms about their appearances left them feeling marginalized and mistrusted. These reported judgements made about their appearances (and subsequent criminalization of their characters) were re-ported to make these young men feel down and (negatively) affected their opportunities to affirm a more positive (social) positioning.

Dean: It annoys me and makes me feel down and bad, 'cos I'm not like that and if someone branded me like a violent antisocial person, it annoys me 'cos I'm not, it really upsets me (Bronze group).

The reported negative impacts on their positive self-belief were further described in terms of society's prejudice against young men. Boys in all groups provided numerous examples of (negative) reactions from the public and police 'for no reason' other than their general appearance.

Rob: If there's vandalism or someone's got beaten up or someone's got stabbed, it's always comes back to teenagers and they cat-egorize you, like stereotype you, if you walk round and you've got a hood on the back of your jumper they'll go, 'Oh there's a hoodie'. They just stereotype you and say, 'Oh he's got a knife, he'll probably be doing some vandalism . . .'
Michael: Yeah 'cos if you're wearing a hoodie and trackies and black trainers they'll [the police] pull you over (Gold group).

These boys' comments indicate some resistance to the judgements made about their chosen styles of dress but also reveal evidence of their perceived powerlessness to act against dominant and negative framings of identity. Here, *power through* these dominant (gendered) discourses was seen to af-fect the boys' perceived *power to* act against judgements made about them and their appearances.

Michael: It puts me on a low, I just walk around acting like I don't care about anything. If I don't feel appreciated, I just walk around thinking what's the point in trying (Gold group).

Other accounts, however, did suggest a different opinion. For instance, some young men expressed their feelings of anger and aggression at being judged as antisocial by virtue of their appearance. Rather ironically, this reported anger and aggression seemed to encourage boys to act in line with these judgements and expectations.

Matty: They look at us funny and you just get really angry, you just feel like turning around and smacking 'em in the head, especially the men.
Researcher: Can you give me an example of what happens?
Matty: If it's an old man then I'll usually go 'What you looking at granddad?' It makes me angry and annoyed 'cos it's not like we do it to them, it pisses you off (Silver group).

Josh: It's like antisocial really. It makes you wanna go beat someone up 'cos you're annoyed, you're angry.
Researcher: What is it that angers you about it?
Josh: It's like nobody trusts you and they think you're gunna like nick a kid or beat up a kid, and we're not like that (Bronze group).

These accounts indicated how boys' appearances, and in particular wearing a hoodie, seemed to (re)affirm a set of gendered expectations of aggressive male behaviour. By challenging these judgements through displays of anger and aggression, these boys seemed to (unknowingly) strengthen the same gendered discourses they sought to resist which, in turn, further spurred their anger and aggression. Thus, these seemingly contradictory elements of young men's expressions of empowerment (in terms of their resistance to the assumptions about their appearances) also appeared to have the effect of re-affirming powerful gendered discourses about young people's appearances.

Talking to others

A final aspect of participants' discussions of being happy tied to the ability to talk to new people. Young people in the Gold group described their experiences of talking with authority figures, including politicians and senior school staff. Members of this group were often involved in efforts to promote the school's positive image within the wider community.

Lucy: If you talk to new people and they like you, then you know you're a likeable person which boosts you and just compliments if people say you're good then that's gunna boost you and makes you feel good (Gold group).

Sarah: I really do think it helps with your whole happiness. I think being able to talk to other people you have to first have confidence in yourself (Gold group).

Young people in the Bronze group also linked being happy to talking to new people but often did so by describing their lack of ability to talk to others. This perceived inability to talk to others seemed to deny them opportunities to develop their confidence, but was also seen as a direct consequence of having no confidence.

Researcher: I don't want to put you on the spot now, but you didn't know me . . .

Kelly: But when I first saw you, I felt like I knew you because when I first started to speak to you, I felt like I knew you, but when I go to other people I don't feel like I know them.

Researcher: But do you know what the difference is? What is it about meeting someone for the first time, like you did talk to me, so what was the difference?

Kelly: Like a person judges you just like that sometimes, and then when you get judged you think, am I that really bad? And then that's when it just lowers you down. . . . Like you, I felt you weren't judging me, that's like why I's thought I've always known you (Bronze group).

This young woman's ability to talk to someone she had recently met seemed to contradict her reported inability to talk to new people but, in so doing, illustrated the ways in which young people's accounts of confidence were relationally framed. In this particular example, having the confidence to talk to a relative stranger was linked to the (nonjudgemental) response received and not because Kelly was simply unable to talk to new people. As I explore in later chapters, members of the Bronze group reported less opportunity to receive such positive and nonjudgemental responses from others, which significantly limited their opportunities for developing a more positive self-belief and thus, feel and be happy.

The chapter thus far has highlighted young people's tendency to describe their health in more positive terms, linked to the various (social) factors that made them feel and be happy. An examination of young people's accounts of being happy has shown how young people's 'belief in the self' is constructed within a complex network of (gendered and economic) social relations. These positive expressions of health indicate a possible starting point for empowerment that is more firmly located within contextual rather than individualized features and, specifically, young people's social positioning in relation to others. I now turn to examine a second key way in which young people reported feeling well through the notion of 'having fun'. The idea of having fun highlighted the ways young people collectively sought to affirm their (social) positioning and set their own agendas in life but which met with some tension from adults' discourses of risk and risk-taking – pointing to some potential competing areas and priorities for health promotion.

Having fun

Young people's tendency to describe their health in more positive ways was also evident in their accounts of what they described as 'having fun' and was closely linked to their descriptions of being happy and feeling well.

Matty: In the summer holidays, we'll go round each other's houses and have a couple of drinks of beer, play on the console and just chill out and have fun.

Luke: Yeah when you get up, ring your mates, you go out . . . you just wander around and have a laugh . . . it's just fun, it makes you feel good (Silver group).

Within the school context, having fun was described as simply 'having a laugh' and 'messing around' and included 'making jokes' and laughing at teachers. Having fun in other contexts was more often described as 'enjoying oneself' or 'chilling with friends' and included activities such as hanging around in parks, playing football and drinking alcohol. Importantly, having fun was described by young people as freeing them from the imposition of control they experienced within the everyday structures and routines of the school environment.

Luke: Tomorrow it's Saturday so if I sat outside my house, I can just put up a chair and sit back, do whatever I want, skate board, bike, play games, whatever. You can just have one day of fun . . . it makes you feel happy and you have a purpose of being on the planet.

Researcher: Do you not feel that on other days then?

Luke: No because on other days you always have something to do, from Monday to Friday we have school, we have to do that and it isn't a feel free sort of way. It feels like your life's being controlled, it makes you feel that your life's stuck in one cycle (Silver group).

The analysis that follows highlights three important meanings young people attached to having fun: *it's just having a laugh, having fun at others, having fun with friends.* These three interpretations of having fun can be linked to empowerment in the following ways. First, young people's accounts of having fun point to a number of creative strategies developed by young people to act in accordance with their own frames of reference. The shared systems of meaning on which these creative strategies were based not only excluded many adults, but also affirmed young people's sense of belonging amongst peers. Second, these collective strategies offered young people opportunities to manage and resist a number of reported (social) pressures linked to their social position. This resistance was, at times, seen to subvert the normal order of the social context in which having fun was experienced. Third, young people's discussions of having fun revealed a more positive discourse (with potentially counter-hegemonic tendencies) to that offered by official health promotion discourses, which often prioritize concepts of risk.

It's just having a laugh

Young people's accounts often suggested that having fun was about 'nothing in particular' and a way to alleviate boredom. Young people across all groups frequently reframed mundane, everyday events as 'entertaining' and seemed to need little stimulus to laugh or find something amusing. Talking in a different voice or walking in a different way, for example, often triggered outbursts of laughter. In this way, young people were seen to create their own innovative forms of entertainment organized around shared systems of meaning.

> Kelly, Sonya and Becky stand outside at lunchtime. Becky starts screeching 'Dr Beeecccccckkks, Dr Beeeecccckkks'. The others stand and laugh at her as she walks around clucking like a chicken. Mr Danner comes over and asks what she's doing. Becky replies 'nothing, it's just having a laugh ain't it'. Mr Danner tells her to be more grown up and reminds her she will be leaving school soon and entering the 'real world'. (Field note)

Examples such as these often left teachers unaware or even confused about why young people were laughing. When questioned about their behaviour by teachers, young people often replied by simply suggesting they were 'just having a laugh'. Observations made in the school context revealed how other teachers responded to these examples more negatively with frustration, often commenting on young people's unacceptable and immature behaviour. Young people's strategies for creating fun seemed to provide teachers with evidence of young people's inability to take things seriously and act responsibly. Consequently, having fun was largely seen by teachers not as a valuable end in itself but as a distraction from the achievement of educational goals. Accounts given by professionals therefore largely prioritized the need to develop young people's maturity and responsibility – an indicator of which was their ability not to laugh at seemingly insignificant things.

However, whilst 'having a laugh' at seemingly insignificant things sometimes met with negative responses from teachers, exerting control over what was seen as 'funny' appeared to add to the fun in two main ways. First, by having fun at nothing, young people felt they were capable of laughing at things adults did not find amusing. This offered limitless ways of having fun in which young people themselves could set the terms of reference for what was considered fun, often to the exclusion of many adults. Adults were further excluded from young people's understandings of having fun as they were often described as 'boring' and largely incapable of enjoying themselves.

Michael: Just 'cos we're kids and we like to have more of a laugh than adults do. We like to have more fun, 'cos adults just sit around and be boring and we like to go out and we just have more fun (Gold group).

Second, lack of clarity surrounding having fun could itself be part of the fun and, indeed, something that young people thought adults could not, and should not, know about. Any attempts to understand what having fun meant to young people seemed to take the 'fun' out of having fun – indicating the value attached to the exclusionary practices that underpinned having fun about nothing. The perceived ignorance of adults was a focal point of reference in young people's accounts. The incapability *and* ignorance of adults enabled young people to demonstrate their own capabilities and authority, as the following interchange reveals.

Researcher: What sort of stuff do you do to have fun?
[Laughter]
Jason: Don't be shy now Luke!
Matty: Kids' things.
Luke: Little kids' things that adults shouldn't know about.
[Laughter]
Researcher: You going to say any more?!
Luke: You might get embarrassed.
Researcher: Try me!
Luke: Just messing around, it's sort of like nothing really (Silver group).

In this way, young people's accounts of having fun can be understood as ways in which they sought to take control over everyday systems of meaning by defining the conditions and setting the parameters for what was seen as funny and, crucially, to the exclusion of many adults. Accounts of 'having fun about nothing' seemed to offer creative ways in which young people could free themselves from adult-imposed conditions in the school context and offered possibilities for (momentarily) shifting the balance of power within the classroom.

Laughing at others

Whilst young people's accounts seemed to suggest having fun was often about 'nothing in particular', jokes and laughter were frequently at the expense of others – in particular, teachers. Laughing at others sometimes resulted in significant disruption to school routine. On several occasions during fieldwork, some of the boys from the Silver group recorded the sound of a fire alarm on their mobile phones and played these back during lessons. Inevitably teachers would respond to the alarms by following fire safety procedures whilst students sat at their desks and laughed at the teacher's response. A further example of the disruption caused by having fun about others was seen at a school music event.

> We sit on the back row, a student begins to sing and Nathan says loudly, 'Oh my god, she sounds like a screaming cat'. He begins to mimic her singing much to the amusement of others. When the performance is over they all clap, cheer, stamp their feet and call out 'encore'. Mrs Payton looks to the back row and appears unimpressed as she indicates for them to be quiet. Several members of the audience also turn to see what is happening. . . . A second young performer starts to sing, but then suddenly shouts 'fuck' across the microphone and walks off the stage. The young people burst out laughing as the teacher facilitating the performances attempts to defuse the 'outburst'. She seems embarrassed and the others laugh loudly. Mrs Payton then comes over and sits with us for the rest of the event. (Field note)

On this occasion, having fun by laughing at others disrupted the performances and added to the discomfort of the teachers hosting the event. The reaction of teachers and the (largely adult) audience highlighted the ways in which adults (in this context) often perceived young people's expressions of having fun as evidence of their lack maturity and respect for others. However, young people viewed such events as 'just having a laugh', and they were largely found to be so amusing because of the (negative) reaction from others and, most notably, the potential to cause disruption and subvert the normal ordering of events.

Having fun with friends

Being with friends was a third theme in young people's accounts of having fun and again highlighted the value placed on the *relational* aspects of developing a positive self-belief. Having fun with friends included 'hanging out' in local parks and the town centre, watching television, chatting, going shopping, playing football and drinking alcohol.

David: I just love nights like going out.
Matty: And you don't need to be in at a certain time.
Luke: I just love it when there's one day you can sit and relax and there's no rules . . . because you spend every day in like a ruled world and there's not hardly anything you can do, and then you've got one free day, like what Gaz said about going out on Friday night and

do whatever you want, you feel better, you feel like you can do something with your life (Silver group).

Drinking alcohol and smoking were seen by some respondents as part of having fun with friends, these practices being positively linked to young people's desires for greater freedom. Young people's discussions also revealed a gender difference in the health-related practices of boys and girls (cf. Dixey *et al.* 2001, Rugkåsa *et al.* 2003, Shearer *et al.* 2005, Nichter *et al.* 2006). Some boys, notably those from the Silver and Bronze groups, reported a preference for smoking cannabis. Whilst some research has suggested that boys' use of cannabis and other illicit drugs can be seen as expression of the need to be 'tough' and 'hard' (see Courtney 2000, Haines *et al.* 2009, deVisser and McDonnell 2013), the boys in this study discussed how smoking cannabis could be 'funny' and made them 'feel free' and relaxed from any worries and pressures in their lives. In particular, smoking cannabis was valued as a means of pacifying aggression rather than asserting themselves. Accounts of smoking cannabis can be seen here as a way in which some boys actively sought to resist, and potentially 'free' themselves from, the demands of more traditional gender norms linked to dominant forms of masculinity (cf. Knight *et al.* 2012, deVisser and McDonnell 2013, Oliffe *et al.* 2013).

Gary:	It's just like when you're round your mates and they're having it [cannabis] they're always happy around you.
Matty:	You don't think about anything, you just think about good things you don't think about the bad things. . . . Everything's just clear, you feel just like free.
Researcher:	And that's a good thing?
Matty:	Yeah, 'cos sometimes especially when you're pissed off with someone you'll go out with your mates and have a joint and then you feel better, you'll just chill out, you don't worry about things (Silver group).

Similarly, drinking alcohol was reported as helping some boys (particularly in the Gold group) to feel free, relaxed and have a good time with 'the lads'. Importantly, drinking alcohol was not discussed in terms of 'laddishness' and the pursuit of sexual conquest (themes often highlighted in the literature, see Connell 2005 and Haenfler 2006, for example) but was largely described as an opportunity to 'chill out' and relax with friends.

Nathan:	You just feel good about yourself, 'cos when you're with your mates and you're drinking, you can't ask for much more really, it's just a laugh. . . . We had all-nighters like round my mates, it's awesome, just listen to music, get drunk, have a laugh, it's just like quality times (Silver group).

Although girls were generally critical of smoking cannabis and the use of other illicit drugs, they too openly discussed their positive use of alcohol. Amongst girls in the Gold and Silver groups, drinking alcohol was reported to make them feel and be more sociable. Drinking alcohol was further described as making them feel confident, which helped them better negotiate social encounters and, importantly (in opposition to traditional forms of femininity), to assert themselves within these settings.

Gina: It's easy to talk to people and get to know people if you're drunk (Gold group).

These positive links young people made between their health-related practices and the factors they identified as supporting their self-belief raise some important questions about the assumption often made in official health discourses that processes of individual empowerment straightforwardly translate into positive health outcomes. Drinking alcohol and smoking cannabis were not discussed by young people as being particularly problematic for their health but instead were viewed more positively as offering pleasure and freedom from the imposition of control in their everyday lives (cf. Bogren 2006, Järvinen and Gundelach 2007, Tutenges and Rod 2009, Järvinen 2012).

By drawing upon young people's own understandings of health, we can begin to see a possible tension between processes and outcomes of empowerment because young people's accounts of their health-related practices seemed to offer possibilities for empowerment but at a potential cost to their health. Consequently, health promotion efforts aimed at empowering young people (based on the reduction of their smoking and drinking practices) may, paradoxically, hinder the very prerequisites for processes of empowerment identified by young people themselves. This apparent paradox not only raises important questions about the conceptual distinction often made between processes and outcomes of empowerment but further draws important attention toward some of the *unintended* outcomes of the concept that may not be deemed health promoting. These unintended outcomes may, in turn, shape subsequent responses and further the *need* to empower young people according to official discourse. This illustration begins to suggest the relevance of a more dynamic and generative understanding of empowerment in contrast to the more stable continuum suggested in much of the current literature (Nation *et al.* 2008, Pearrow and Pollack 2009).

Young people's discussions of their own health-related practices in terms of pleasure and freedom rather than risk differed sharply from the views of professionals interviewed in this study. Drawing more heavily on dominant health discourses, professionals' accounts tended to frame young people's use of alcohol, and other health-threatening practices, in terms of risks to health.

I think the risk-taking thing, I work with some young people who actually get a buzz from the risk and what might happen, it's not that they're not aware of the risk, but having the risk is part of the buzz. It's like they're getting energy out of taking some risks, whether it's drinking or you know unprotected sex or whatever it is. (Social and Emotional Aspects of Learning [SEAL] Coordinator)

I think in terms of, not just sexual behaviour, just general risky behaviour, if their friends are doing it they'll follow suit because they want to fit in and that can put them in some quite dangerous situations. (School Welfare Officer)

By stressing risks to health, professionals' accounts downplayed the value of young people's friendships and the more social meanings stressed in participants' accounts. As such, young people suggested they had to be careful about how and where they had fun as not only did the police and members of the public automatically assume they were causing trouble, but they also thought that the majority of adults perceived having fun as being synonymous with risky and antisocial behaviour. This reported concern for antisocial behaviour was seen as regulating the contexts available to young people in which to spend their free time.

Josh: They think antisocial like, the way we have fun, like say 'Oh, you're antisocial, don't like you'.
Researcher: Can you tell me about things you do to have fun that might be considered antisocial?
Josh: Probably playing football against a wall, we got done for that quite a bit (Bronze group).
Emily: We use to go up to Treelands, but we're not allowed up there anymore, 'cos the police said we were too loud and if we get caught up there again, like within 48 hours, we're gunna get arrested (Silver group).

Some support for the link between having fun and perceived antisocial behaviour was also found in the accounts given by professionals. Restrictions on young people's use of open spaces were deemed a positive move towards addressing antisocial behaviour in support of young people's health.

Every single child should have an activity that they're involved with and committed to, their life should not just be about hanging out on the streets. I think to be healthy, being at home with their computer consoles or their television, hanging around in the streets, I don't know if that would keep anyone terribly well for terribly long, so a young person in my view should have something that's more than hanging around in the streets and getting involved in drugs and alcohol or antisocial behaviour. (School Senior Management)

However, young people themselves viewed such restrictions not as supportive of their health but as compromising their freedom to act. Adult-imposed limits on young people's freedom ran contrary to the discourse of health found in young people's accounts (which stressed the importance of being happy and having fun). Consequently, young people from all groups discussed how efforts to remove young people from public places were indicators of adults' lack of true concern for their health (cf. Morrow 2000).

Emily: They're not interested, it's not like they're concentrating on us, it's not like they want us to feel good about ourselves, they want us to feel bad about ourselves, so they keep getting the police involved and getting us in trouble (Silver group).

Gina: They don't act like they care even though they like make a big deal out of young people, it's more for their own benefit than it is for ours. Like they're keeping young people off the streets so people don't get irritated, not for our health, they're not thinking that's affecting them in anyway, they're just thinking it's affecting other people, they don't think about us . . . the government themselves don't really make a big deal out of how to make young people happy, they do it of more how to get them off the streets, they don't think about the happiness, just how to get rid of us, like when they hear young people go out on the streets, it's immediately think they're doing stuff. But when I go out I don't cause any trouble, I don't bother people, I'm just trying to be happy and have fun with my friends (Gold group).

Here, an emergent tension between (competing) concepts of risk and empowerment within official health discourse indicates different starting points for understanding young people's health. For example, professionals discussed the value of increasing young people's confidence to reduce the effects of peer pressure but in doing so started from more negative assumptions about what young people *might* do (such as drink or smoke) and sought ways to prevent this. In contrast, young people's accounts pointed to the value of starting with a more positive conceptualization of young people and their health based on what they *actually* did do. According to young people interviewed, these more positive expressions of their health, based on understandings of being happy and having fun, often go unnoticed (or are reframed negatively) by dominant risk-related discourses. Prioritizing risks, rather than health, was seen by young people as denying opportunities for promoting a more positive discourse on their health and one they thought more appropriately reflected the reality of many young people's everyday lives.

Gina: I think they could be less against us and be more like with us . . . they could try and understand us instead of saying to us that's

> wrong, you can't do that . . . like if something bad happens they'll make a big deal out of it, but if they see young people having a good time and having fun they won't take that into account, they won't go 'Oh we should do more things like that because it's helping 'em'. They look at that bad and think how we gunna stop that (Gold group).

A refocusing on the possibilities for health in terms of young people's understandings of being happy and having fun, rather than the problems (in terms of potential health risks), once again raises some important questions about the rather linear pathway to health found in many official health promotion discourses. This more positive focus lays the foundations for a more dynamic conceptualization of empowerment whereby positive understandings of health can be seen not only as a catalyst for empowerment in line with young people's perspectives but also a product of processes of empowerment themselves.

Conclusion

In this chapter I have analysed young people's understandings of health in line with their own frames of reference. Young people's definitions of being happy highlighted a tendency to describe their health in positive terms – often linked to the importance of developing a positive self-belief. Examining young people's discussions of a positive self-belief highlighted the various (social) factors that made them feel happy in terms of *knowing I can do something, looking good,* and *talking to others.* These findings point to a number of important contextual, rather than individual, prerequisites for empowerment.

Young people's discussions of having fun similarly pointed to their preference for more positive expressions of health and highlighted the different strategies they developed to act in accordance with their own frames of reference. These collective strategies enabled young people to take control of, and sometimes subvert, the normal social order – revealing some possibilities for collective forms of empowerment. Examining young people's accounts of having fun, however, also raised some important questions about whether empowerment promotes positive health outcomes in line with official health discourses – highlighting too some possible *unintended* outcomes arising from processes of empowerment.

6 Not feeling well
Being judged and misunderstood

In this chapter I examine young people's accounts of 'not feeling well'. Specifically, the analysis that follows takes forward some of the contextual and relational framings of young people's health revealed in Chapter Five. By doing so, I aim to bring to the fore some of the varying ways in which different forms of power (*power to, power over, power through*) operate to (negatively) affect young people's experiences of health – highlighting too some further tensions for understanding the concept of empowerment.

Being judged

Young people's accounts of 'not feeling well' were heavily dominated by reports of being judged by others, including their peers, adults and society more generally. Young people in this study made repeated references to how they were often misrepresented and misunderstood by others and in particular, by adults. These judgements were believed to compromise the potential for a more positive understanding of young people and their health and often differed from many of the priorities set out in official health discourses.

Researcher:	What things might stop you from feeling well?
Carl:	Stereotyping.
Researcher:	Can you say a bit more about that?
Carl:	Teenagers are labelled tracksuit-wearing, knife-carrying chavs who take drugs, drink, smoke . . .
Researcher:	And how does that impact on you then?
Carl:	It makes you feel down 'cos I'm not like that, but I get labelled it, it's really not nice (Gold group).

Researcher:	What does not feeling well mean to you?
Michael:	When people like think of us, like degrading us, like if someone's saying stuff about you that can put you down. That has a massive impact on me, when I feel like everyone's judging me. It just makes you feel low, it's like I just wanna do nothing in life (Gold group).

'Young and dumb'

Young people's accounts of being judged seemed to suggest that 'being young' was seen by many adults as synonymous with 'being dumb'. Across all groups, young people talked about how adults treated them as if they were thick, stupid and immature on the basis of their age alone. At school, comments made by teachers often drew attention to young people's lack of knowledge, maturity and ability to understand and follow instructions. In this context, observations made in the school setting seemed to reflect wider social norms about young people's perceived developing competencies and capacities (cf. David, Edwards and Alldred 2001, Milstein 2010). In particular, interactions between members of staff and students indicated that the former frequently drew upon dominant developmental and protectionist discourses (James and Prout 1997, Mayall 2002) – and often made reference to young people's (lack of) maturity. These developmental assumptions about young people's abilities were seen by participants as restricting their opportunities and *power to* decide and act for themselves. Consequently, young people frequently described how many of their views and suggestions went unnoticed, or were negatively sanctioned, because of (adult) assumptions about their perceived maturity and capacity to act responsibly.

Josh: They [teachers] think we're too young, they all think you're thick. I think 'cos we're young they think we're thick and we don't know stuff, that it won't get stuck in our head, but it does (Bronze group).

Gina: I think people just think that when people are younger they can't make decisions and they're not old enough to decide for themselves and have their own opinions because they're not mature enough yet to make their own decisions. I think it's just summat that people are accustomed to, thinking that young children can't go beyond a certain point of thinking (Gold group).

At times young people in the Bronze group, and some members of the Silver group, appeared to buy into these developmental assumptions as they too described themselves as being 'thick' and 'stupid'. In particular, members of the Bronze group made repeated references to being 'dumb', 'picked on' and not listened to because they felt they were deemed incapable of handling academic requirements or making (positive) decisions for themselves.

Sonya is upset because she hasn't heard back from the college. She seems convinced that she won't get accepted and begins to tell me how everyone in her life has put her down by calling her 'stupid', 'thick' and a 'retard'. She says, 'I'm just a retard so what's the point? If people tell you something often enough you start thinking and believing it'. She is close to tears as she continues to tell me about how her parents, brother and teachers put her down for being 'thick'. (Field note)

Arguably, these self-criticisms could be seen to provide some support (and impetus) for promoting the (individualized) forms of empowerment that seek to increase young people's self-esteem and confidence (see for example Tones 1998a and b, Zimmerman 1990, 1995). However, despite often doubting their individual abilities, at other times these same young people showed considerable insight into the various structural factors (and specifically the school cohort system) that seemed to deny them important opportunities to show what they could do given the opportunity.

Kelly: I reckon they think we're dumb . . . but they make us sound like that 'cos they put us in this half, it's like the way they've done it now it's making us think we're all dumb basically (Bronze group).

The school's positioning of young people according to their abilities not only signalled to these respondents that they were largely believed to be incapable and incompetent but was also seen by these young people to limit their opportunities to show their abilities and prove otherwise. Young people from the Bronze group in particular were highly critical of the school's cohort system and for what they saw as the positive and preferential treatment of the Gold group.

Kelly: They all pick on the [Bronze group] basically; they have more respect for the [Gold group] than they do us. . . . They think that we're like dirty trash basically; they've just thrown us away because we're down on grades. But it's not our fault why we's thinking like it, it's basically their fault 'cos of what they've done, they should have let people done all choices what they've thought had been right (Bronze group).

These young people's reports of the perceived preferential treatment received by young people in the Gold group were not, however, confirmed by accounts given by members of this latter group, who similarly described how they felt they were judged as being immature and incapable of making (positive) decisions for themselves. In this way, whilst young people thought there were differences between the groups, a commonality of perspectives was observed. Here, the school system seemed to create a potential barrier to more collective forms of empowerment as young people were relatively unaware of the close synergies in their perspectives and, in particular, the social conditions they mutually felt positioned them as being relatively powerless to act within the school context.

The marginalized (social) positioning experienced by those in the Bronze group not only signalled these young people's awareness of their relative lack of *power to* act in the school context but also pointed to evidence of their (critical) engagement with the exclusionary effects of power and, specifically, the impact this exclusion had on their self-belief and feelings of worth. Despite such insights, this awareness was not seen to trigger the forms of critical action that might prefigure collective forms of empowerment (cf. Ruston 2009). Instead, young people in this group seemed to suggest there was little point in trying to challenge teachers' perspectives of them.

Examples of 'giving up' often played out as flouting school rules, such as turning up to lessons late or skiving (playing truant), wearing incorrect uniform, smoking, swearing, eating, drinking and using mobile phones during lessons. Examples of these young people's apparent disregard for school rules, however, seemed to confirm teachers' low expectations of the Bronze group and supported beliefs about their inherent lack of ability to act maturely and responsibly. In this way, young people's resistance to the school environment (as one possible starting point for empowerment) seemed to have the (unintended) effect of supporting and reinforcing the very discourses which positioned young people as being incapable of acting responsibly – which, in turn, set further limits to the possibilities for their empowerment.

In contrast to the (negative) accounts given by members of the Bronze and Silver groups, teachers and other school staff often commented on the more positive possibilities the cohort system facilitated, such as ensuring 'appropriate' support was offered to the different groups. Because teachers and professionals working in the school understood the cohort system to be a positive structure, they read the Bronze group's (dis)engagement as evidence of their individual failure to know what was best for them. On the basis of these perceived individual failings, school staff often reflected low expectations of these students.

> The teacher tells me it is a waste of time coming into the lesson as no one does anything, he says 'these students are at the lowest end of low and I'm just here for crowd control really and to manage things'. The teacher does not give them any work and there seems to be nothing set for the lesson . . . the students simply play games on the Internet. (Field note)

Further observations made during fieldwork, however, offered powerful counter-evidence to these (low) expectations of these young people. During some lessons, members of the Bronze and Silver groups were seen to produce extensive amounts of written work and participated in discussions on topical concerns. Furthermore, young people's accounts of their personal lives exemplified the ways in which these young people challenged the idea that they were immature and irresponsible. The personal circumstances and home lives of some young people revealed insights into their capabilities to self-manage very challenging situations. These circumstances included dealing with the complexities of absent parental figures, families with drug and alcohol dependency issues, and parental involvement with police and social services. In contrast to being seen as immature and irresponsible, the caring responsibilities placed on these young people could be argued to demonstrate their ability to act as mature and responsible beings as they took on, and dealt with, a number of difficult and demanding personal circumstances.

For example, Kelly – a girl from the Bronze group – described the responsibilities she had at home, which included caring for both her parents who had drug and alcohol dependency issues in addition to looking after her five younger siblings. Managing these responsibilities whilst trying to meet the demands set by the school was seen by Kelly as a testament to her personal strength to manage not only her own life but those of others. However, in the school context, Kelly's contributions (and those made by other young people) to the lives of their families were largely unknown or unrecognized.

Kelly: I look after people, like my dad and my brother. . . . That's why I find it hard to do homework at home and teachers telling me off saying I'm not doing this, I'm not doing that, but if they lived in that house for a week they wouldn't last there for that long (Bronze group).

Examining young people's resistance to the assumptions made about their lack of ability and maturity to act responsibly revealed how young people's relative *power to* act can be understood, not as an individual deficit, but as a product of a social context, and in particular a school system that appeared to reflect and reproduce wider social norms about young people's (in)capabilities (cf. David, Edwards and Alldred 2001, Milstein 2010). Here, the starting point for forms of psychological or individualized notions of empowerment may not be located within the development of young people's (deficient) personalities or particular psychological attributes but instead must begin with a more thorough analysis of the operation and effects of *power through* dominant (developmental) discourses that serve to (re)produce the (disempowering) structures that set limits to some young people's opportunities to demonstrate their *power to* act (particularly in the school context). The importance attached to a refocusing on what young people can do, rather than what they are deemed incapable of doing, once again came to the fore as young people underscored the value they gave to being recognized for their achievements and contributions – a theme I explore further in subsequent chapters for its potential contribution to young people's health and health promotion.

Despite young people's frequent criticisms of being judged as relatively immature and incapable, comments made by some teachers provided some alternative perspectives to young people's accounts. In the school environment, individual discussions with staff pointed to the possibilities for a more positive view of young people as they underscored opportunities for respondents to make personal choices. These more positive examples illustrated the operation of a coexisting (and potentially competing) discourse about young people and their abilities to act. In contrast to the accounts provided by young people, at times teachers were seen to encourage young people to make informed and 'responsible' decisions – particularly with respect to their behaviours and health-related practices.

> I think because as they're getting older they have more freedom to make their own choices about their lifestyle, I think that's when they start to have to make decisions for themselves with things like substance misuse or sexual health; they'll start focusing more on their choices. (Learning mentor)

This discourse of 'choice', however, often presented itself as a contradiction to young people who further pointed to examples of times when they were asked to be more 'adult-like' and act responsibly but then denied opportunities to do so because they were considered to be too young and immature. Young people frequently discussed times when they thought they had to make important decisions about their future but were then told by teachers and parents they were not old enough to make decisions about what they could do in their own time.

These restrictions seemed to be guided by dominant protectionist concerns as accounts given by adults suggested young people were likely to make decisions that would contravene their best interests. Here, notions of empowerment at the first dimension of power as the *power to* act were seen to be shaped by the ideological effects and operation of *power through* dominant discourses which come to define what young people in this context were considered capable of doing.

Sarah: We're kids and why can't we just be kids? It's like they tell us not to grow up too fast and we can't do stuff, but then they try and make us grow up by like saying you've gotta be more mature. It's like they're contradicting themselves.
Researcher: So how are they telling you not to grow up too fast?
Sarah: With our parents we're not supposed to be growing up too fast, but then, in another direction we've got all the teachers saying we've gotta chase our [exams], we've gotta think about what we wanna be when we're older, but we're supposed to still be kids and they won't let us do anything. It's just so confusing; they just contradict themselves all the time (Gold group).

This contradiction was not only challenged in young people's discussions of their abilities to make positive decisions for themselves but was also heavily criticized as evidence of adult hypocrisy. Young people often pointed to the discrepancies between what adults said they did and what they were seen to do (see Spencer 2013c).

> Zara and Lizzie told me they saw some of the teachers smoking at lunchtime. They found this funny and told me how the teachers would be in a lot of trouble if they did say anything. They criticized the teachers for being 'so hypocritical'. (Field note)

Concern about adult hypocrisy was further evident in the (contradictory) messages relayed in health education sessions, which often prioritized notions of informed choice and individual responsibility (see for example Department of Health 2010b). In the school environment the promotion of choice-based discourses existed in competition with the view that young people were largely incapable of making informed decisions for themselves and often as a consequence of their susceptibility to 'peer pressure'.

Young people's (critical) accounts of the developmental discourses that define and position them as being largely 'incapable' appeared to exist in some tension with official health promotion discourses that promote the idea of a rational autonomous being (cf. Katainen 2006). Consequently, in their efforts to display their capabilities and resist judgements made about being 'young and dumb', young people's accounts often revealed how they themselves drew on notions of choice. Here, young people's discussions on a range of (health) issues highlighted the importance of *choice* in relation to their health-related practices. Indeed, young people often demonstrated their knowledge of, rather than their ignorance about, the implications of taking up health-related practices deemed harmful to their health (cf. Baillie *et al.* 2005, Katainen 2006, Abbott and Dalla 2008).

Aaron: I think I should be able to make my own choices about drinking and smoking and sex, it should be my decision, 'cos who else's business is it really if I wanna smoke, it's me, it's harming my body. If I wanna smoke weed, I'm not making other people do it with me, it's their choice if they wanna do it (Bronze group).

Claire: You should have the decision yourself rather than somebody saying . . . there are smokers but they know the risks, if they still wanna do that then let them, it's their choice (Gold group).

Although young people's preference for the notion of choice appeared to challenge developmental assumptions about their lack of maturity and capabilities, this resistance came at the expense of acting against official health promotion messages that stipulate people should largely abstain from health-threatening practices. Whilst teachers and adults more generally seemed to view young people's resistance to health promotion as evidence of a lack of maturity and ability to make informed healthy decisions (thereby confirming the message of the competing developmental discourse), young people's accounts of acting contrary to official health discourses stressed their ability to make healthy decisions according to their own frames of reference (i.e., by resisting the judgement they saw as negatively affecting their health).

In this context, young people's accounts of the choices they made regarding their health-related practices could be argued as evidence of an expression of their empowerment and *power to* act against adult opinion as they actively sought to resist the judgements made about their maturity and capabilities. In this way, judgements made about young people's immaturity and assumed inabilities to act responsibly triggered some young people's 'choice' to act against adult judgement. Far from being incapable, young people's accounts suggested how engaging in risky health-related practices offered some young people opportunity to display their *power to* make informed decisions according to their own frames of reference and crucially, by doing so, attempted to challenge *power through* dominant developmental discourses that define young people as being largely incapable and immature.

These illustrations of young people's displays of resistance to dominant developmental discourses similarly point to the potential significance of some of the *unintended* consequences of young people's empowerment. These unintended consequences, in turn, can be seen to reinforce the very impetus for empowerment as evidence of young people's *power to* make health-related choices (and resist dominant health promotion messages) may trigger a further 'need' to empower young people in order to reduce the risks to their health stemming from their health-related practices. This more dynamic operation of the concept points to the relevance of a more generative understanding of empowerment, whereby different forms of power intersect to produce differing outcomes for young people's health – a crucial point I take forward in Chapter Eight.

Being bad

One further important aspect of being judged described by young people tied to the idea that being young is equated with 'being bad'. Reflecting widespread (adult) anxieties and recent media reports about a disengaged and troubled youth (Kelly 2000, 2003, Messias *et al.* 2008), young people across all groups described how they felt adults, and society more generally, readily and uncritically assumed that all young people were inherently 'bad people'. The tendency to pathologize and problematize young people was heavily criticized by respondents as evidence of a lack of trust and respect (cf. Valaitis 2002, Messias *et al.* 2008).

Rob: I feel judged, as teenagers we're judged by everyone, they stereotype us, they're a teenager, they're doing summat wrong. I think with our age they sort of pick you out like you're the culprit, you're the bad person (Gold group).

Carla: They just think we're all bad and they don't respect us. They tell us we gotta respect them, but they don't talk to us or respect us and I really think they need to have more respect 'cos we're not bad. . . . Old people can be so horrible to you, most of them just think you're bad and don't talk to you or like talk down to you as if you don't matter . . . they just treat us like we're all bad (Bronze group).

Sustained attention toward young people's 'bad' behaviours was frequently reported by participants to (negatively) affect young people's everyday lives and undermined the more positive discourse found in young people's own accounts of health (i.e., in terms of being happy and having fun). Of particular importance were young people's descriptions about how the lack of trust and respect arising from these negative judgements made them 'feel down', 'unhappy', and 'worthless'. Young people made links to their positive self-belief as they described times when they themselves questioned whether they were indeed 'bad people'. This self-questioning illustrated some of the (negative) consequences such problematizing discourses held for young people's own understandings and experiences of health.

Sarah: If you walk down the street they [adults] look at you as if you're scum, and that just does absolutely nothing for you as a person, it makes you feel like if they all think that of me then it makes you feel like you are . . .

Researcher: Some of the reactions actually make you feel like you're scum?

Sarah: Yeah you feel like you are, it's *really* bad for your self-confidence. . . . It knocks you, it irritates me, and really annoys me, 'cos they don't know me, or what kind of person I am (Gold group).

Lucy: I don't think that adults or people in society realize that when they put this image of teenagers all being yobs that they're actually affecting the teenagers. I know that we just live with it as a way of life, the fact that people expect us to be bad and horrible. We shouldn't have to feel like that.

Researcher: When you say 'you feel it', how does it make you feel?

Lucy: It makes you unhappy, it makes you feel worthless, you're like why should I bother, if all they think of me is that. It does make you feel bad (Gold group).

In their discussions, young people in this study not only drew particular attention to popular media images of 'problem teenagers' but also revealed how dominant constructions of youth as a time of risk (negatively) impacted on their experiences of health. Specifically, by promoting and reproducing these images, the media were heavily criticized by participants for portraying unrealistic and negative stereotypes of young people. Respondents interviewed in this study thought that many adults had assimilated these (negative) images, which, in turn, they believed affected their everyday interactions and relationships with adults. Across all groups, participants provided numerous examples of times when they felt they had received negative and even hostile reactions from members of the public (cf. Morrow 2000).

Sarah: They just think kids are a load of yobs. . . . They've been so use to this image that when they actually meet someone that stereotype's still there in the back of their heads, there's still that thing saying this person's a yob, this person's a *classic* young person (Gold group).

Nathan: They hear so many bad reviews on the news – 'teenager mugs old woman'. The other day this lady dropped her bags and I was, 'Do you wanna hand?' And she was, 'No I can do it myself'. She thought I was gunna do summat, but I'm not gunna hurt anybody, I'm not like that. It's 'cos of all the reviews on teenagers, they just think bad of us (Silver group).

In their discussions of these incidents, young people often linked prevalent media representations of a troubled and problematic youth to dominant health education discourses. Attention to public health priorities such as teenage pregnancy, smoking, drinking alcohol, drug use, and antisocial behaviour were described by respondents as (unfairly) reflecting and promoting a negative image of young people's health and likewise believed that such portrayals influenced young people's everyday interactions with adults. The assimilation of these official health discourses by adults was described by young people as affecting their actions and opportunities to help others and, in particular, restricted their freedom to go about their everyday lives – as Claire's detailed account illuminates:

Claire: I've got a really younger brother, there's a huge age gap, I was 12 when he was born and my sister was 16 and we're in town and she's pushing the pushchair, and he went to grab something, and this old lady went, 'Can you not control your kid?' That's not my child, it's my mum's.
Researcher: And what was her reaction then?
Claire: She was like 'Oh sorry, I thought you were one of those'. That's what she said!
Researcher: How did that make your sister feel?
Claire: She won't push the pushchair because of it. Why should my sister be made to feel like that when it's not her fault? It's just not right. It's happened to me as well, my brother was 2 so I was about 14 and I was in the shop and this old lady was like, 'Do

you know how to control your child? If you don't why did you
have it?' I didn't, it's my brother, do you not understand that?

Researcher: Did you say that?

Claire: No, because I didn't feel that I should, why should I explain myself . . . that made me feel really bad 'cos I felt,
god have I done the wrong thing, should I not have come
out? Why should I not be allowed to do stuff with my
brother? I'm against it, all of this stereotyping. . . . Like a
lot of teenagers are seen to have all these things wrong
with them, but again it's hardly any of us (Gold group).

These examples, and many others, were discussed as evidence of adult
discrimination towards young people. In particular, young people described
the forms of ageism they experienced – highlighting times when they believed parents, teachers and others stigmatized and excluded them on the
basis of their age alone.

Steve: I think older people are ageist to young people. They think
they're chavs who are gunna knife them . . . when you see an
old person they give you a funny look.

Nick: It's like once I got the impression when I went into the shop
that like if I'm buying something the person is treating me
with suspicion.

Carl: Yeah they think you're gunna rob, like if you walk into a
shop, if someone comes in my age, like a group of them, oh
they're all gunna rob (Gold group).

Rob: I think its discrimination. I just think it's stereotyping just because we're that age, they just sort of categorize you. We're
sat there doing nothing and then you get the police come
along and start checking you, searching you, just because of
the age we're at. If there was a group of men walking along
or whatever, they might stop them, but they wouldn't search
them. It's just the age that you're at (Gold group).

Of particular importance to young people was the suggestion that the
current (political) attention toward antisocial and risky behaviour did not
acknowledge the more positive expressions of health found in their own accounts in terms of being happy and having fun. The failure of official health
discourses to resonate with the more positive aspects of young people's everyday lives not only reduced the saliency of health promotion messages,
but by marginalizing these positive aspects, a focus on risky health behaviours worked, rather paradoxically, against the promotion of young people's
health according to their own frames of reference. Young people's examples
of resistance to health promotion can be therefore understood not simply as

their disregard for the achievement of positive health but as an active challenge to the negative stereotypes that young people themselves felt compromised their own experiences of health.

Power through these official health discourses was also seen to guide parental opinions and decisions. In their accounts, some young people described the ways in which parents would draw upon dominant negative images of young people to set rules and boundaries. For example, parental concern about teenage pregnancy, drunken and antisocial behaviour influenced curfew times and regulated young people's peer relationships. These restrictions were again seen by these young people as being particularly unfair and as an index of parental mistrust.

Kirsten: I don't get much choice. They're too strict. My parents are on my back for everything, they don't trust me.
Researcher: Why are they always on your back?
Kirsten: I don't know really, they just tend to think that I'm a bad person.
Researcher: Why do you say they think you're a bad person?
Kirsten: They don't like the friends I hang around with, they think they're a bad influence. . . . They think I get proper drunk every weekend. They just don't trust me (Silver group).

Reports of parental use of the same negative discourses that young people saw as adversely affecting their health not only compromised young people's positive beliefs in themselves but set limits to some young people's *power to* negotiate and influence boundaries at home, including opportunities to exercise choice and *power over* their own lives. For instance, Kirsten (a girl from the Silver group) described in detail how she was not allowed to stay out after 4 in the afternoon. According to her account, she felt this curfew was linked to her father's concerns about her assumed involvement in binge-drinking and drug use, or her potential risk for getting pregnant. Although this young woman dismissed her father's concerns as ridiculous, she ultimately felt she had little choice but to agree with the rules set down by her parents.

Kirsten: I think it's just 'cos teenagers are like that, they [parents] stereotype me.
Researcher: Can you tell me how they stereotype you?
Kirsten: They just think I'm gunna get like a pregnant teenager, but I'd say I'm not ready yet. But my dad thinks I'm just gunna sleep with anyone and get pregnant (Silver group).

Young people's discussions about their parents' lack of trust appeared to reflect wider (public) concern for young people's inherent wildness. The general expectation of young people's unruly behaviour was thought to provide little incentive for young people to be good. Whilst for members of the Bronze group (and some members of the Silver group) attention given to disruptive acts triggered episodes of swearing or messing about, young people in the Gold group thought there was little point in trying to challenge these expectations of young people's behaviour – often suggesting they could not be bothered to question the perspectives of teachers or other adults.

Michael: I'll do something good and people don't see it and then I just think what's the point, I won't bother then . . . it just makes you feel low, it's like I just wanna do nothing in life, there's no point (Gold group).

Sarah: It makes you feel why bother? They're gunna think that no matter what you do, so why bother trying to change that? (Gold group).

Furthermore, and rather ironically, the sustained negative attention on young people's lives was also seen by some respondents to provide the impetus to act in the very way such judgements expected. Paradoxically, young people's accounts pointed to the possible ways in which a focus on health promotion itself can prompt the very risky behaviours it aims to reduce (cf. Crossley 2002).

Andy: I think people judge you a lot, you get looks from people, when you walk into a shop and the people at the counter will be watching you, so that makes you feel like why? If they like think of us that way, why don't we just do it, why don't we just do what they think we're gunna do. It makes you feel if they're judging us, what's the point in acting any different (Gold group).

Lucy: It does affect you because you think what's the point in trying to be nice if they've got this perception of you, what's the point in trying to be anything different. I might as well just go out and get drunk and drink on the street because that's what people think we should do (Gold group).

Despite being highly critical of the negative attention given to young people's lives, respondents themselves were seen to (re)construct and reproduce these problematizing discourses in two main ways. First, young people's accounts drew attention to the behaviours of the risky bad Others (see also Spencer 2013c). Whilst often aware of being judgemental, young people sometimes drew upon official health discourses in their discussions of other young people's (health-related) behaviours.

Lucy:	Even I do it to other young people and that makes me feel bad as well.
Researcher:	Do you know why you do it to other young people?
Lucy:	Because of the image that people have. I'm sure all those young people in tracksuits and hoodies are lovely people, but because the media present that image of them . . . I don't wanna call them chavy but they are, no 'cos it's stereotypical, but they have that chavy label and the fact that they smoke and they drink like every single weekend and get drunk (Gold group).

Whilst this construction of the risky younger Other enabled some young people to dismiss the relevance of health risks to their own practices, these discussions also indicated a tension for the development of collective notions of empowerment (Spencer 2013c). Specifically, these accounts of other young people's bad behaviour were seen to divide different groups of young people, marking out the 'good' from the 'bad'. The symbolic boundaries created by different groups of young people were supported by the school's cohort system as each group felt that other groups received preferential treatment for either being good or for being bad.

| Lisa: | I think the naughty kids they're allowed to do much more than we are, and we don't get praised for being good. Like they get to do these stupid trips and the rest of us have to stay at school and because they're naughty they get to do more. I don't agree with that, I think that's really out of order. It's so unfair, because they don't deserve it (Gold group). |

These divisions were seen to reduce possibilities for young people to recognize the *commonality* of their perspectives – a key prerequisite identified in the health promotion literature for collective forms of empowerment (Laverack 2009, Wiggins 2011). Here, the more divisive consequences of *power through* dominant problematizing discourses (reproduced within the school's cohort system) ultimately limited the possibilities for young people to collectively challenge the discourses they themselves felt had significant impacts on their health. Crucially, in order to come together collectively, young people would need to recognize their common position with other young people and their shared status of 'being young'. However, not only was this status of being young challenged by young people for its negative connotations, but rather paradoxically, by buying into and adopting this shared identity, respondents needed to place themselves in alignment with, rather than resistance to, the very status that they sought to challenge (Spencer 2013c).

A second way in which young people's accounts supported the reproduction of problematizing discourses of youth was through examples of individual efforts to resist such discourses. Young people discussed times when they had individually questioned and challenged the accuracy and authority of teachers, parents and the police. However, these challenges were most usually seen by adults as examples of young people 'answering back', which ultimately resulted in young people getting into more trouble. Young people's resistance was not only limited by the ways in which adults drew upon problematizing discourses in their responses to young people's questioning but also how these challenges (re)affirmed dominant beliefs that young people were inherently bad.

Andy: It makes you angry and they suspect you even more because you're getting jippy with them.

Researcher: What happens there then?

Andy: We're just standing there and then they get more firm, 'You have to leave now otherwise we're gunna get the police involved'. So that makes us even more angry because we're voicing our opinion by saying that we're not actually doing anything wrong . . .

Researcher: But if you say anything back to them . . .

Andy: You're digging a hole. They're just gunna pick on you even more 'cos it's more like that stereotype (Gold group).

Gina: They see a group of people out at night and 'cos they see so much bad, they think that everyone whose doing good is also doing bad, so they give you the wrong opinion which makes you more against. 'Cos if someone comes up to you and you're doing nothing wrong and they say to you you're doing something wrong it gets you angry doesn't it? It makes you get aggressive, you think why should I be told that I'm doing something wrong when I know for a fact that I'm not (Gold group).

Despite claiming they had done nothing wrong, when young people answered back or questioned adults or the police, these challenges to adult opinion and authority seemed to confirm the adult suspicion that some young people had something to hide or were in fact doing something wrong. In this way, young people's less powerful positioning in relation to adult authority limited opportunities for effective resistance (cf. Aggleton 1987) as they often felt they has little choice but to agree with the actions of adults and the police or risk further sanctions. Whilst at times verbally challenging and defying adult sanctions, young people were often seen to act in line with the enforced proscriptions on their lives. Rather paradoxically, young people's concordance with the directions of adults and the police provided some potentially powerful counter-evidence that young people were in fact, not bad.

Rob: You've just gotta do what they [adults] say otherwise you'll get done, but it's like they just stereotype you and categorize you and we just gotta do what they say (Gold group).

Conclusion

This chapter has focused on young people's accounts of not feeling well and by doing so has revealed the various ways in which participants felt frequently judged by others and, in particular, by adults. Examining young people's accounts of being judged highlighted the different priority areas young people held for their own health and were further linked to a number of coexisting and competing discourses that appeared to shape the possibilities for their empowerment. Evidence of young people's resistance to, but also assimilation of, these competing discourses pointed to some young people's *power to* act according to their own frames of reference but were also seen to reinforce the consequences of *power through* these discourses. Of significance are the ways in which any possibilities for collective forms of empowerment were limited by the more divisive effects of these problematizing discourses that appeared to leave young people unaware of their shared experience that, if more systematized, might lay the foundations for challenge to these discourses.

In Chapter Seven, I take forward these (health-related) concerns identified by young people by examining the various ways young people sought to challenge these more negative discourses on young people's health and, crucially, to bring about change in line with their own perspectives and priorities for health.

7 Young people's priorities for health promotion

In the previous two chapters, the analysis focused on young people's own understandings of health and what they considered to be some of the key challenges to their health. Drawing on young people's priorities for health promotion, in this chapter I examine the various ways in which young people sought to influence matters of most concern to them and bring about change in line with their own understandings of health. Young people's accounts highlighted three important principles for health promotion: listening, choice and respect. These three concepts are examined here to illuminate the meanings they carry for young people and the implications they may hold for informing concepts of empowerment.

Having a voice

Listening to young people's views was seen as an important starting point for challenging many of the widespread (negative) assumptions about young people's health. In their discussions, participants signalled the importance they attached to listening as a precursor for bringing about an advanced appreciation of young people's lives and challenging some of the inequities they reported to experience as a consequence of their nonadult status.

Melissa: Young people don't really have much of a say, the school don't really talk to us about what we want, and like government because they're so high up. I think if people are making decisions about young people then obviously young people have gotta be involved (Silver group).

Gina: They should just listen more and not be so judgemental about the age and maturity level. . . . The way they treat young people is like they don't have an opinion, but I think they should listen more (Gold group).

Despite stressing the importance of 'having a voice', young people frequently expressed their frustration at the apparent inability and unwillingness of adults to listen to their views (some exceptions are discussed later in this chapter). This reported failure to listen to young people seemed to be linked to the different ways in which respondents felt judged by others. Specifically, young people's accounts illustrated how the reported widespread adult mistrust of young people effectively served to exclude their opinions from entering into (and influencing) discussion.

Charlotte: Because we're children, they won't listen to us.
Lucy: It's because they have this bad perception of us. I just think they feel that we're not worth bothering with and that our ideas aren't like valid (Gold group).

For members of the Bronze group, and for some young people in the Silver group, teachers' failure to listen was further linked to their (marginalized) position within the school. In their accounts, these young people once again signalled the perceived preferential treatment of the Gold group, believing that teachers and the school more generally listened to and valued the perspectives of young people in this latter group.

Josh: They listen to all the people who [are] doing good in school, like the people who are really good, that's what they listen to. They don't listen to us lot. . . . We don't get any say in it (Bronze group).

However, young people in the Gold group similarly reported that they felt their views were dismissed by teachers. Recognition of this commonality of experience by young people themselves seemed to be once again compromised by the separation created by the school's cohort system, which limited opportunities to foster a collective understanding amongst young people themselves.

Lucy: Because that image of them you wouldn't go up and talk to them because you're scared of them and that's a horrible thing to say because they're young people just like me. But the fact that they've made young people seem like that, even young people are scared of talking to other young people (Gold group).

Young people across all groups also described times when they thought offering their opinions would get them into trouble. Specifically, opportunities to (positively) contribute to school discussions were thought to be limited (and even denied) when young people expressed a contrasting perspective to that offered by adults. Respondents described the ways in which offering an alternative view could be reframed as 'wrong' by teachers and parents.

Researcher: If you had the opportunity to say 'We think this is most important . . .'

Sonya: [*interrupts*] No 'cos then we'll probably get told off . . .

Researcher: Why would you get told off?

Sonya: Because we'll probably get done for speaking our minds wouldn't we?

Researcher: You'd get told off for speaking your mind?

Sonya: Yeah because, if we say we don't feel like we're being paid attention and the [Gold group] are being paid more attention, and we feel like all you do is stick up for the adults, then we'll probably just get told off even more (Bronze group).

Rob: You don't get believed by adults because of your age and because you've got your own opinions to things. I think young people speak their minds, that's the thing that gets us into trouble a lot (Gold group).

The powerful role adults had in validating or rejecting young people's point of view illustrated the ways in which young people's *power to* express their opinions was bounded by the ways in which teachers (and other adults) exercised *power over* the views deemed permissible within a given context. Permissible views were further compromised by having to fit within *power through* dominant ideologies, which governed what was determined as an (adult-defined) accepted view. In this way, opportunities to have their opinions regarded were not seen to occur when adults agreed with young people's views, but the reverse – young people had to agree with an adult-expressed perspective.

Researcher: Do you feel you can say what you think?

Wendy: It depends if I'm reasonable to them [parents], then I probably could.

Researcher: What do you mean by 'if you're reasonable to them?'

Wendy: So if I said something they would have to agree with me, *no*, I would have to agree with them to say what I think (Gold group).

Rob: If they say what is your opinion on something, and then you say something they don't want to hear, you can get told off for it because it's not what they want to hear.

Researcher: So when they ask you for your opinion what do you think they expect?

Rob: Exactly, I think they just expect along the lines what they wanna hear . . . they don't like your opinion. They're sort of telling you what they're supposed to tell you, but it's not always how it is in real life (Gold group).

In these discussions, young people (particularly members of the Gold group) further described the ways in which parents often supported the perspectives of teachers. Events at school were often reported back to parents who then disciplined young people for disruptive or unruly behaviour. Young people themselves discussed the unfairness of these actions and the failure of their parents to listen to their own perspectives on these events. Respondents reported the special difficulty they had in understanding why their parents would uncritically accept the perspectives of teachers as being the 'truth'.

Michael:	Like the teachers are adults and we're just children so they think, 'oh well if that's what an adult's saying', then that makes you believe them more because they reckon adults are more trustworthy than children. It's alienating for us because you feel like they trust adults more, just 'cos they're an adult.
Researcher:	Why would they trust the adult more?
Michael:	I reckon it's 'cos they think we're still not properly socially developed (Gold group).

Rob:	I called a teacher, I didn't call him 'Mr' [*laughs*] it's true, and he rang home and my mum made it out to be the biggest thing ever when I haven't said anything.
Researcher:	Did you try and say that to her?
Rob:	Yeah, but she just sort of sides with them. 'Cos they're an adult and they trust them more than they trust us (Gold group).

These accounts indicate how parental alignment with the perspectives of teachers was linked to notions of (mis)trust arising from the social category of age. Young people described how being trusted was tied to the achievement of maturity, and because they felt most adults seemed to equate being young with immaturity, young people thought they were automatically mistrusted and their perspectives dismissed. Here, *power through* these dominant developmental discourses not only limited young people's opportunities to feel and be trusted but also fuelled and sustained mistrust of young people as incidents reported by the school provided parents (and other adults) with evidence that young people really cannot be trusted. Although some exceptions were noted (discussed later in this chapter), many young people thought they could do little to challenge this mistrust because of the dominant belief amongst most adults that the perspectives of young people were invalid and not to be trusted.

Despite young people's reports of a lack of action taken by the school, some potential mechanisms for listening to young people were found within the school environment. At times during fieldwork, school staff were seen to support and advocate discourses of participation by encouraging young people to express their opinions during lessons and engage in forums such as the school council and school parliament.[1] These opportunities were particularly valued by the school for positively supporting young people's involvement, offering opportunities for young people to influence matters of most concern. However, despite the school's positive intentions to facilitate student participation, these (adult-imposed) mechanisms to effect change were heavily criticized by some young people for three key reasons, with some important implications for understanding the concept of empowerment.

First, some young people reported little interest in participation forums, suggesting they were happy with their lives at home and school and thus did not wish to change things in their lives. These particular accounts further underscored young people's preference for a more positive perspective on their health and lives.

Aaron: I am quite happy with the life I have at the moment. There's nothing wrong with it and so I don't really want to change anything (Bronze group).

Emma: I'm quite happy with the way things are. . . . There isn't really much that I want to or that I feel that should be influenced because I'm happy with everything in my life (Gold group).

These accounts illustrate the possibility that participation may not be something that all young people want and, paradoxically, how the concept of empowerment must also hold possibilities for young people to choose *not* to want to participate or change anything in their lives. Whilst these positive reports of some young people's lack of desire to effect change could be read as an indicator of a form of 'false consciousness' or 'disempowerment' (thereby prompting the impetus for Freirean forms of critical consciousness raising), these accounts also reflect what some young people considered to be the more positive reality of their everyday lives.

Here, the key tension for empowerment comes from the concept's prime focus on the conditions of young people's disempowerment. Although empowerment is overwhelmingly presented as a positive approach to young people's health, the concept implicitly begins with a focus on young people's negative experiences of risky health practices and potential powerlessness – both of which young people in this study frequently contested. In this way, by highlighting experiences of disempowerment, the concept runs counter to the more positive discourse young people themselves used to describe their own health – thereby playing into the very (disempowering) discourses that young people saw as adversely affecting their health. Consequently, young people's concern for a refocus on who they were and what they did (rather than what they were deemed incapable of doing) not only signalled their preference for a more positive starting point for health promotion but can be also understood as a challenge to some of the original theoretical underpinnings of empowerment.

A second criticism made against notions of participation was seen in the suggestion that forums to include young people were believed to be 'targeted' towards (and therefore only accessible to) certain individuals – notably members of the Gold group, and specifically the 'good' students in this group. Although teachers suggested that (in theory) these forums were open and accessible to all students, in practice many young people felt only those students with a good academic record were able to access and participate on these committees – a finding widely echoed elsewhere in the literature (Alderson 2008, Wilson 2009, Wyness 2009, 2012).

> *Pete:* Well, I'm one of the students out of god knows how many, they're not exactly gunna listen are they? They brought out the student council and that don't really do much. . . . They're supposed to make students sit down and make decisions, how to make the school nicer, changing rooms, toilets better, but they never actually take into consideration what everyone's said (Silver group).

Observations made during fieldwork also provided evidence of the inconsistency between the participatory intentions of these forums and the exclusionary processes that operated in practice. Members of the school council typically included students with high academic potential and whose parents were governors of the school. Although teachers suggested there were ample opportunities for young people to influence matters at school, these opportunities were only available to a few 'good' students.

A third criticism made against forums such as the school council focused on the potential of these participation mechanisms to create and sustain a pretence of listening, but were ultimately considered ineffective at taking young people's view seriously to bring about change – often referred to as *tokenism* in the participation literature (Hart 1997, Thomas 2007). Young people discussed how they felt the school council would not listen to their ideas and how 'nothing gets done'. Once again, young people attributed this lack of action to the (lack of) value given by adults to their ideas.

Efforts to listen to young people were therefore thought to merely serve to give the impression of listening rather than offering any meaningful power sharing. Although adults perceived such examples as evidence of young people's participation and *power to* act, accounts indicate how young people thought adults ultimately retained *power over* participation agendas in order to sustain an illusion of 'empowerment'. Adult *power over* participation agendas was ultimately linked to the effects of *power through* dominant discourses, which served to disqualify young people's contributions.

> *Steve:* It's just to give the impression. It's just a way to think that students help but they actually don't make a difference.
>
> *Carl:* There's the student parliament, but I don't think anyone goes because they know nothing gets done (Gold group).

Ian:　　　It's just so young people can feel like they're doing something when they're not. I don't want to sound like really sceptic, but it's just like a cover, they just wanna seem they're like taking the views of the pupils into account when they're actually just doing what they want (Gold group).

These particular examples of participation efforts aimed at empowering young people can be thus further seen as a means of 'giving power' rather than young people 'taking power for themselves' – thereby undermining the more bottom-up principles of empowerment (Labonte 1993, Laverack 2009).

Although some respondents were critical of the ways in which participation agendas created a false impression of young people's *power over*, this awareness was not seen to trigger critical action. Instead, young people's accounts pointed to their feelings of ambivalence and lack of action as they reported little incentive to express their opinions or attempt to effect change.

Simon:　　It puts you down, you just think why bother, they're not gunna listen so why bother saying anything to try and change anything (Gold group).

Despite this ambivalence, a closer examination of young people's discussions revealed something of the importance young people gave to 'having a voice' compared with 'making a difference' – with some further important implications for the distinction made between processes and outcomes of empowerment. The suggestion that forums such as the school council merely gave the impression of listening was often substantiated by a lack of evidence of any change to the school environment. This reported lack of change in outcomes provided young people with the evidence that their views had not been listened to or taken seriously – which was ultimately the point of most concern for these young people.

Andy:　　I'd like to change the outcome, but I'd be happy enough just getting my opinion across and knowing that other people have heard and respected my opinion and tried (Gold group).

Rob:　　　At the end of the day it doesn't matter if they don't accept your opinion, as long as you get your opinion across.
Researcher:　So does it matter to you if you don't change things then?
Rob:　　　No, as long as you've put summat forward (Gold group).

Although these comments may support the suggestion that some young people were relatively happy simply putting forward ideas rather than changing outcomes, these accounts also pointed to young people's concerns about influencing matters that extended beyond (structural) issues within their immediate environment. By stressing the importance of expressing their opinions, young people's accounts point to their desire to challenge *power through* dominant norms that were seen not only to limit opportunities to have their views listened to but also to determine the value and integrity of their perspectives. Here, expressing their opinions was not directly valued for its potential to facilitate young people's *power to* or *power over* participation mechanisms but for the possibilities for challenging *power through* those dominant discourses that young people believed disqualified their perspectives from reaching and influencing mainstream discussion and that they saw as negatively affecting their health. For some young people, prioritizing the process of empowerment was in itself an important outcome that signalled to them that their opinions had been duly regarded and valued.

Having a choice

A second way young people sought to influence things in their lives was revealed in their discussions about the importance of choice. Notions of choice were particularly valued by young people as an expression of their freedom and *power to* act according to their own frames of reference. The notion of choice was closely tied to young people's discussions about the willingness of adults to listen to young people's perspectives. Of interest was the idea that having a choice made young people felt they were being included in matters of importance to them.

Luke: We should all be able to make a choice, 'cos everyone has a choice, a say in this world, everyone should have a say in what happens, it makes you feel good knowing you've got a choice (Silver group).

Rachel: We haven't really got much choice.
Sian: Yeah and if you like try and speak they ignore ya [teachers].
Kirsten: They try tell you what to do and what's right and you shouldn't do this.
Melissa: Yeah they don't let you speak out.
Sian: If you're in a meeting, and then they speak and then they don't let you speak, they butt in halfway through (Silver group).

Despite indicating a positive preference for the notion of choice, young people's discussions more often pointed to their lack of choice to act according to their own frames of reference. Participants often stressed the ways in which they felt many adults controlled their freedom and *power to* exercise choices. These restrictions were seen to be closely linked to some of the ideological effects of *power through* dominant discourses that defined not just young people's perceived (in)capabilities but also the agendas around which young people were given opportunities to exercise *power over*.

Luke: Most of the times I don't feel I can go out much because my mum gives a time limit, so I don't have much freedom to go out and that feels as if it's controlling . . . she's worried I'll go out and like get into trouble (Silver group).

This reported lack of choice appeared to be closely connected to young people's (social) positioning as those who were not yet adult. Imposed limits to choice were thought to exclude young people from more 'adult' agendas and what young people termed 'the real world'. In their accounts, young people once again reiterated the widespread mistrust for young people and how this mistrust effectively served to limit the choices available.

Luke: We're excluded, we're not trusted in the world, we're not really wanted until we get to a certain age and then we're let in. It's like we don't feel that we have a say or a choice in our society and we're being controlled because we don't get a say (Silver group).

In particular, *power through* dominant discourses was seen to structure the inequities young people felt they experienced as a consequence of their age. Young people often gave examples of age limits that effectively prevented them from engaging in a number of choice-based practices valued by young people such as joining the local gym, buying alcohol, learning to drive and exercising a right to vote. These statutorily imposed age restrictions were thought to be unjustly based on (negative) assumptions of what it means to be a 'typical teenager' – an image some respondents wished to challenge and change.

Luke: Everything is over the age of what we want it to be, just 'cos the adults decide we'll be stupid and mess around, they don't think we can be mature enough to do something, they put age limits for everything.

Matty: People try rule our lives even if it's not our parents, everybody's ruling our lives . . .

Luke: You should never ever control someone else's life 'cos you're making decisions for someone else when you wouldn't like it, you would really hate it if someone did that to you, stopped you, made you do everything you didn't wanna do, but that's what they do to us (Silver group).

Of particular concern to respondents was the suggestion that these limitations to choice (compounded by the failure to listen to young people's views) provided evidence of adults' (and society's) lack of care about young people. This perceived absence of care was seen not only to affect young people's feelings of (self) worth but was also reflected in some young people's critical engagement with the suggestion that adults had the power to control their everyday lives. Young people's use of the term *choice* was not valued simply for its potential to demonstrate their *power to* and *power over* their own lives but was tied to an overwhelming desire to foster young people's inclusion as valued members of society. For young people involved in this study, exercising choice was seen to offer the potential to shift *power through* those dominant (problematizing and developmental) discourses they believed excluded them from influencing matters of concern.

Luke: We may be younger, but we have a mind of our own and because they don't trust us about what we say, it makes us feel that we are inferior as in we shouldn't be here, that we don't have a right and we should just been in a kids' planet or they should put us all on the moon. We live in an adult world, but we're still kids and they don't want us to be kids, they're trying to get us to be adults before we are adult. We're being forced to do both, but they're not treating us as if we are proper adults. . . . We are kids and we know what we need to do, but they treat us as if we don't know and we should be in a completely different set of rules to the adults, they're treating us un-human, because they're treating us like we're a different race, it's like we're two different races because we have two different sets of rules which is sort of un-human towards us (Silver group).

Luke's detailed account of feeling excluded highlights the negative impacts this form of power has for young people's feelings of (self) worth and opportunities in life. Here, some respondents' engagement with the socially located conditions of inequity signalled young people's critical, rather than false, consciousness. However, this critical engagement once again seemed to do little to trigger overt action to bring about change as predicted in much of the literature on empowerment (Laverack 2009, Wiggins 2011). This lack of action questions the widely held idea that critical awareness of power inequalities is the starting point for empowerment. Young people involved in this study, whilst often engaging with the effects of dominant power regimes, more often stressed their relative lack of influence to change existing arrangements and dominant systems of meaning. In particular, challenging the social construction of age was thought to be limited until they were themselves were considered adult. Here, young people's accounts of effecting change seemed to indicate their acceptance of, rather than resistance to, the existing social order.

Simon: I'm just seen as a kid really, I don't think I could influence anything (Gold group).

Stephen: I don't really think you can change things to be honest, not at this age you can't really influence things (Gold group).

The disenfranchising effects of the social category of age on young people's opportunities to exercise choice were further reproduced within the school cohort system. Members of the Bronze group often drew attention to the ways in which the school structured choices available, with implications for future career aspirations. For instance, subjects including business studies and sociology were not available to students in this group. In addition, these young people were entered for examination papers that would only enable them to reach a minimal grade. These limitations were seen by members of the Bronze group as being particularly unfair and based on assumptions about their perceived academic incapability to succeed. Young people in the Bronze group discussed the implications of these imposed restrictions for their future life chances and pointed to the ways in which *power over* their own lives was defined by a school system that seemed to reinforce the wider age (and potentially class-based) inequalities experienced by this group.

Kelly: I think the school is in charge of us group's life, but they're not in charge of the higher group's because they basically just put all their choices what we should go for. But we should've picked our own choices, and let us have a go and if we don't think it's right for us then we should be able to move into another choice, but they just don't let us. To me I reckon they think we're just dumb. . . . Everything's like, you can't do what you want these days, it's like you've gotta do what people say. The higher groups got all their choices ain't they? What they wanna do in life, they've all got them choices and then like when it comes to us we don't have a choice. . . . I haven't got a choice over anything (Bronze group).

In contrast to the perspectives given by members of the Bronze group, teachers viewed these restrictions as evidence of the school's support and care for members of this group. By only offering options deemed appropriate, school staff thought they would not be setting these young people up to fail. Under the guise of protectionism, teachers' accounts not only justified the school's *power over* these young people's lives, but also revealed how developmental assumptions about young people had potential consequences for other forms of social inequality, including those linked to future occupation and class position.

The protectionist approach taken by the school was heavily criticized by young people in the Bronze group not only for contributing to their marginalized (social) positioning but also for drawing attention to their perceived incapability and incompetence rather than a more positive focus on what young people might be able to achieve given the opportunity.

Kelly: If they least give us a try of what we wanna do maybe we might do well. . . . If they like give us more encouragement and like let us do things what we think we're capable of. Like they say people make mistakes, well we should learn from our mistakes what we choose, and now they haven't, now they keep saying that we're pushing you to do this work 'cos we want you to get higher grades, but it's like pushing us down because we know we're not gunna get a high grade (Bronze group).

These accounts given by members of the Bronze group pointed to the effects of a lack of choice on their future life chances and the potential ways in which the inequalities of age *and* social class intersect to shape the opportunities available. More significantly, these young people's discussions not only highlighted the ways in which the social category of age was seen to produce its own forms of inequality but also how assumptions on the basis of age were effectively used to mask and justify the reproduction of other forms of inequality, such as those linked to class position.

Despite young people's overwhelming concern about the lack of choice they experienced, two key contradictions emerged in their discussions that are worthy of closer examination. First, accounts given by some young people did offer clear examples of times when they felt they had made choices for themselves. In these discussions, young people often drew upon notions of responsibility and, as Kelly described, the idea that 'making a mistake' sometimes had positive outcomes for future decision-making. Here, exercising choice was particularly valued as means through which young people could resist the assumptions stemming from developmental frameworks and demonstrate their responsibility to make decisions for themselves.

Dean: If you're told not to do something it just makes you do it really. It gives me more responsibility knowing I'm allowed to drink 'cos it makes me feel a bit, you know, like I have a say in the matter (Bronze group).

In some ways, this focus on demonstrating responsibility could be seen as some young people's alignment with, rather than resistance to, developmental discourses that have a tendency to prioritize young people's (lack of) ability to act in more responsible ways. However, young people's accounts more often underscored the positive ways in which they thought they were able to negotiate and set boundaries for themselves. Opportunities to exercise choice not only offered young people *power to* make decisions and take *power over* their own lives, but in exercising choice young people can be seen to challenge the *power through* dominant discourses that defined young people's perceived abilities to make responsible decisions for themselves.

More positive examples of times when respondents felt they made decisions for themselves were evident in some accounts of their relationships with parents. Members of the Gold group (and some members of the Silver group) often discussed the ways in which they negotiated rules and boundaries at home – suggesting some possible class-related differences in the negotiation of boundaries with parents (cf. Bernstein 1977, 1982, 1990, Devine 2004, Devine *et al.* 2005). Of particular interest was the idea that exercising choice did not necessarily imply young people wanted to act against parental (or adult) opinion.

Lucy:	I think that my mum and dad have always had the mentality of I can do whatever I want, like within reason obviously, but because they've always brought me up with if I want to do something they'll pretty much let me do it.
Researcher:	What does 'within reason' mean?
Lucy:	Well I wouldn't ever ask to do something like, 'Can I go and tattoo my face', no I wouldn't because I've always been allowed to do things . . .
Emma:	You set your own boundaries . . .
Lucy:	Because I think some people, their parents say they have to do this, it makes them want to do things, rebel against it. But because I've always been brought up with the 'you can do whatever you want', like they obviously care, but 'we don't mind what you do', that I don't push it, so I don't really have anything to rebel against (Gold group).

These accounts given by some young people suggest that exercising choice was not purely an individualized process of decision-making but a means of facilitating collective dialogue *with* parents as they negotiated boundaries together. Of particular importance to young people was the suggestion that negotiating boundaries with parents provided evidence of parental trust and respect for their perspectives and actions and thus contradicted their previous reports of the lack of trust they experienced.

Nathan:	Like my mum and dad have a say, because obviously like any parent would do that, like caring and stuff and that's good. I'm not like overruling my parents because I have so much respect for them so it's just like if they say like 10 or something, I'll be like yeah sure. . . . They don't mind if I'm out like clubbing or summat, they're just like, 'Oh make sure you've got your house key because we'll be in bed by the time you get back' (Silver group).

A second contradiction found in young people's discussions linked to times when they described imposed limits to their choices in a more positive manner. Some young people talked about wanting some limits and did not always express a desire to make choices for themselves.

Hayley: If you don't have boundaries you're gunna think that when you go out into life, it doesn't matter, you've got to have boundaries 'cos it teaches you in life and gives you responsibility (Silver group).

Gina: I mean my parents sometimes stop me from going out, but then I sort of side with them on that one because I know that if they let me out too much I won't get into the habit of doing work. But if I'm inside, I'll do something like revise and its helps me to achieve (Gold group).

These more positive discussions of boundaries also revealed the importance young people attached to feeling valued and included as a positive contribution to their health. In particular, young people in all groups suggested they wanted to feel included in matters affecting their lives and wanted support and guidance from adults when making decisions. Of interest was the idea that boundaries signalled to young people that parents (and other adults) cared about them and what they did. Parental care was therefore given as a worthy reason for any restrictions to young people's choices.

Rob: I think parents do it for your best interests, it might not seem like it, if they're strict on you . . . but in the long run you'll benefit from it . . . because you've got some of these parents that really don't care, they let their child go out, be naughty, go out, drugs, drinking and all that. But then you got like my parents, the stricter ones, they'd give you a certain time to be in. They're only doing it for your best interests. . . . I think it gives you a better upbringing, it gives you a better know how (Gold group).

Whilst these accounts may again imply young people's alignment with paternalism and their assimilation of 'best interests' concerns operating within developmental discourses, the existence of rules and boundaries provided some counter-evidence that challenged young people's own suggestions that adults seldom cared about them. Here, some limits to young people's *power to* and *power over* can be seen to support a positive shift in *power through* dominant discourses as limitations to choice provided important counter-evidence to the suggestion that adults did not care.

Treat us with respect

One final aspect of effecting change in support of young people's own ways of seeing health focused on the importance of respect (cf. Valaitis 2002).

Respect was valued by young people in this study not only for its potential to support the development of a more positive self-belief but because respect offered an important starting point for challenging the negative discourses young people saw as adversely affecting their health. Here, young people's accounts reinforced their preference for being seen for who they were and not what they were assumed to be.

Researcher: What do you think it would mean to you to be trusted and respected?

Carl: I'd feel a better person 'cos it's like, oh I'm actually being treated finally like for whom I am, not for who like a minority of people my age are (Gold group).

Young people's use of the term *respect* drew particular attention to the more positive aspects of their lives and was intricately linked to their own understandings of health as they described the importance of being recognized for doing well to their experiences of being happy. Being positively recognized was seen as an opportunity to foster a greater understanding about young people and what they could do when given the opportunity.

Michael: To be recognized that I've done something good is a really good feeling, but half the time they [adults] don't trust us with our own lives and it just really brings you down. . . . Until we're adult they won't appreciate the stuff we've done. We wanna be recognized for the things we do, that makes us feel good (Gold group).

'Saying something positive' about young people was suggested to be an important starting point for redressing the negative focus that was usually given on their lives. In particular, developing opportunities for young people to show their strengths, rather than highlight their assumed deficits, was closely linked to other concepts found to be of importance to young people's opportunities to effect social change, such as notions of listening and choice.

Melissa: I think they should talk to you as younger people and see how we feel about things, I think they should actually ask us how we feel about life and things that's happening around us.

Researcher: Why's that so important?

Kirsten: Because they always do stuff to benefit older people and not younger people . . . they need to think that we got better ideas and respect our ideas (Silver group).

Luke: I just feel we should have more freedom for them to listen to us, and they don't tell us what we are able to do they just tell us what we can't do. Give us the opportunities to think about these things, instead of, 'Don't go hurt someone, rob a car, don't sit in front of the TV, don't drink, don't smoke, it's bad for you'. . . . It's saying something positive, instead of just keeping it negative. . . . It's all negative, 'Don't do this, don't do that', but they don't say, 'Why don't you go out and do this?' (Silver group).

Discussions of respect were also seen to challenge widely held (adult) views that young people were disrespectful to others. In these accounts, respondents drew attention to some of the more positive things they did for the community and reiterated the value of developing a positive understanding about young people. In contrast to professional concern about reducing risky behaviours, young people's accounts illustrate the contributions they made to the lives of others and offer positive suggestions on how young people could be included as valued members of society. In particular, young people signalled the importance they gave to being seen and valued as (younger) *people* and not as 'youths'.

Dean: I think they need to focus more on the good sides, like what we do for the community, it's like we're equal as the next person, we're just the same, we're still members of society. . . . I think tolerance and a bit more open mind towards young people (Bronze group).

Researcher: What's wrong with the name 'youth club'?
Lucy: It's just kind of like you're being labelled. It makes me think of a place where they just shove you because you're 'youths'. It sounds so bad, it sounds like it's where all the trouble-makers go . . . they just make us sound as if we're so different and bad that we have to be shoved into a 'youth centre' (Gold group).

Challenging negative discourses of 'youth' and using the lexicon 'young adults' was not only seen as an important shift towards respecting young people but also pointed to respondents' engagement with the ways in which different terms describing their nonadult status (such as *youth*, *adolescents* and *teenagers*) contribute to marginalization. Here, fostering inclusion requires moving beyond involving young people in matters of concern to effect a redefinition of discourses surrounding 'youth', including the particular terms young people believed (unfairly) defined and positioned them as being inferior by virtue of their age alone.

In some ways, young people's discussions of respect could be seen as evidence of their assimilation of ideas akin to the recent political focus on respect in the United Kingdom (Respect Task Force 2006) and wider related discourses of citizenship circulating within the school environment. In the school context, display boards, citizenship lessons and discussion topics in assembly and tutor time often focused on promoting young people's respect for others. Although promoting respect might suggest a more positive approach taken by the school, this more recent political attention to the notion of respect appeared to stem from an assumption that young people were disrespectful to others – a starting point that was frequently challenged by respondents.

Michael: It just makes you think how ignorant some older people can be, do they have no respect at all for young people? They should be respecting young people more, not treating them as [if] they were all naughty five-year-olds.

Researcher: How do you think that would help young people?

Michael: Because I think most of all we just wanna be treated with the same respect adults demand from us. They want respect from us which half the time they don't give back (Gold group).

This more negative understanding of respect as the need to reduce instances of *dis*respect was not only seen to influence a number of resistance strategies, such as answering back to teachers, but differed from the understanding of respect present in young people's own accounts. In contrast to the unidirectional notion of respect often presented by teachers, whereby young people were charged with the responsibility of showing respect to others, young people's accounts indicated a more reciprocal understanding of the concept.

The potential value of this reciprocal approach for promoting young people's health was particularly evident in the few positive examples given by young people of times when they reported they had felt respected by others. In these accounts, some opportunities for shifting power relations emerged. For instance, certain teachers were reported to be respected by young people. When young people were questioned further about these teachers and their relationships with them, their accounts linked the respect they held for these teachers to the level of respect they themselves felt they received. In particular, their accounts underscored the importance they attached to being seen for whom they were, as they warmly described how some teachers had taken time to get to know them and in doing so, showed respondents they believed in them.

Rob: Like Mr Woods because he listens to your opinion instead of bossing you around. . . . I think he's like taken time to know each of us, to know us individually. He sort of knows how to treat each of us, he knows us individually and he's taken time to get use to us and show us respect and that's why we're all doing so well now because we have respect for him . . . he's respecting how we feel and showing us he's there for us and showing that he believes in us (Gold group).

Carl: Mr Stevens like my PE teacher, he's the best teacher around, because he's like so respectful to the students so he gets respect back (Gold group).

Likewise, when reflecting on their participation in this study, respondents highlighted their preference for a more reciprocal notion of respect. The broadly ethnographic approach to the research necessitated prolonged engagement in the field. The sustained time spent with young people was in itself seen by respondents as a mark of respect for who they were – in contrast to judging them for what they might be. This approach was thought to provide young people in this study with a valued opportunity to share and demonstrate what they thought were the more positive realities of their everyday lives. This mark of respect for their perspectives was reported by participants to enable their more meaningful participation in the study.

Carl: Like this, 'cos you're taking your own time to come and talk to us and you're not doing it on your own like points of view, it might just be better, you're not stereotyping me, so I feel comfortable so I'm showing you respect if you know what I mean? So if people actually took the time to get to know us, something like this, then they might actually see what we're really like and what really matters (Gold group).

Despite stressing the importance of *reciprocity*, young people provided numerous illustrations of occasions in which they felt they received negative (and discriminatory) reactions from adults. These reactions revealed how young people's preference for more reciprocal notions of respect could inadvertently fuel disrespect between adults and young people.

Researcher: So what happens when you feel you're not respected?
Carl: In a way you try like annoy them, 'cos they're like annoying me so I wanna annoy you, 'cos you're making me frustrated I wanna make you frustrated, it's like a vicious circle really (Gold group).

Pete: They wanna be respected, but then they're not giving us respect.
Researcher: How do you think that could change?

Pete: Well rather than always grassing us up and complaining about us, come and have a word with us. . . . What you find, residents on the streets, they come and give you crap basically. We just throw it straight back at them and then that's where it comes back as all these youths aren't very polite. Whereas if they's to come along, speak to us with respect first, rather than just gobbing off, then we're not gunna gob back (Silver group).

Discussions of the lack of respect young people experienced and their responses to this not only highlighted how dominant power relations were reinforced but also revealed a significant tension within existing conceptions of empowerment. When asked how respect for young people could be fostered within society, respondents repeatedly referred to the actions of adults that effectively served to marginalize and exclude them.

Dean: I wish you could just hold your head up high walking through where you live, because of not the way you dressed because you know, you don't get branded with the same eye that some people are so, you could like hang your head high. These days it's hard to do that 'cos you get marked and you get shunned. . . . It's like a no-win situation, if we're not respectful we get stick, but if we're respectful we just get shunned (Bronze group).

Carl: It's just the same like with older people and teenagers, we're the ones that will always get in trouble 'cos they're older, but they're like the least respectful people out of all of them. Some of the way they talk to kids and it's just like we don't stereotype them . . . they're so disrespectful (Gold group).

These accounts signal how any possibilities for empowerment based on young people's preference for the notion of respect must also closely examine the perspectives and actions of the adults that ultimately make young people feel undervalued and excluded from society.

Nathan: I'd just like to see an older person, like walk past us and not feel intimidated, not feel like they're gunna get beaten up. That would make me feel really good, they just make it all sound as if we're just having unprotected sex, getting wasted, getting in fights, smoking weed, taking drugs. We're not all bad and they all think that we just get drunk, shag the first thing that comes along, do drugs. It would be nice to know that they're not actually thinking of us like that. I'd like them to present us in a better way and let us have fun with our friends without the police having a go at us (Silver group).

Crucially, young people's accounts pointed to the role of adults, government and media in challenging the (negative) conditions and discourses they saw as working against the promotion of respect between young people and adults. In particular, young people wanted others (especially adults) to offer a more positive discourse on young people's health and alter the structures that were seen to reproduce negative discourses about young people. Possibilities for bringing forward a more positive discourse on young people based on a more reciprocal notion of respect were, however, closely linked to the perceived willingness of adults to begin the process of listening, trusting and respecting young people and provide more opportunities for young people to demonstrate the positive aspects of their lives and the many contributions they made.

This dependence on adults' perspectives and actions demonstrates not only how the effects of *power through* dominant discourses limited opportunities for young people's inclusion but also (and in contrast to current theorizations of empowerment) how the starting point for any possibilities for empowerment may not begin with young people themselves. Young people's accounts here challenge the suggestion that empowerment is exclusively a bottom-up process. Instead, these accounts point to the important role played by those in positions of power, such as adults, in providing and facilitating the necessary preconditions for young people's empowerment. However, in doing so, a fundamental paradox exists because those in a position to facilitate possibilities for young people's empowerment were also seen to be part of the problem working against opportunities for empowerment. The different perspectives seen in accounts given by young people and adults thus raise critical questions about how empowerment may be facilitated by those who were also seen to (re)produce the very discourses young people saw as adversely affecting their health and that they wished to challenge. Here, the concept of empowerment remains problematic when young people look to, and are dependent upon, the willingness of adults to challenge negative (mis)understandings of young people and thereby (re)construct a more positive discourse on young people's health.

Conclusion

In this chapter I have examined some of the different ways young people sought to influence matters of most concern to them. Listening was seen to be a key prerequisite for fostering young people's inclusion and, in particular, redressing the effects of *power through* dominant discourses which come to define the validity and integrity of young people's perspectives. The notion of choice was also valued for enabling young people to exercise *power to* and *power over* their own lives and, in doing so, challenge *power through* dominant discourses that position them as being largely incapable of making (positive) decisions for themselves. Finally, the value of a more reciprocal exchange of respect between adults and young people was seen as being fundamental to developing a positive appreciation of young people and what they do – offering some potential to shift power relations and foster a more positive discourse on young people in support of their health.

Developing this positive discourse, however, highlighted a number of tensions for the concept of empowerment as young people looked to adults to develop a deeper and richer understanding of their lives and instigate positive social change. Here, a fundamental paradox emerges whereby the actions of those in a position to facilitate the prerequisites for young people's empowerment were also instrumental in limiting possibilities for change. Whilst adults were seen by young people as key instigators of change, young people's dependence on adults to shift their perspectives on young people raises crucial questions about whether empowerment can be understood as exclusively a bottom-up process.

8 Empowerment and its relationship to young people's health[1]

This chapter focuses more closely on the concept of empowerment and its possible links to young people's health. I start by revisiting some of the theoretical tensions outlined in Part One of the book in order to address more firmly three key issues in the current literature on empowerment and health. First, I identify some of the assumptions that emerge from the conceptual distinction made between individual and collective notions of empowerment. The analysis that follows examines these assumptions more fully and considers the implications from research findings for both individual and collective approaches to empowerment. In doing so, the discussion challenges existing theorizations of empowerment that suggest there is a relatively linear continuum from individual to collective action.

Second, I further trouble the distinction often drawn in the literature between processes and outcomes of empowerment. The discussion illustrates how processes of empowerment can in fact result in variable and indeterminate outcomes. These unintended effects, in turn, affect subsequent responses (both those of adults and young people themselves), creating both possibilities for and limitations of young people's empowerment.

Third, as I have argued in previous chapters, current uses of empowerment often fail to work with an adequate theorization of power. This omission has a tendency to oversimplify the relationship between power and empowerment as it affects young people's health. Drawing on Lukes's (2005) tripartite perspective of power, in this chapter I aim to develop a more theoretically informed conceptualization of empowerment and thus, advance understanding of the concept's relationship to, and relevance for, young people's health. Crucially, this chapter seeks to offer a more dynamic and generative conceptualization of empowerment than hitherto articulated in the literature, informed by a multidimensional perspective of power.

A new conceptual framework for empowerment as it relates to young people's health is proposed based on two distinct but interrelated understandings of health. The first, more dominant perspective is premised on the normative frames of reference that inform official health discourses; the second reveals some of the alternative discourses on health that emerged from young people's own accounts. These two understandings of health help to inform six conceptually distinct forms of empowerment that capture and synthesize individual, structural and ideological elements of power that differentially (and sometimes inconsistently) shape the possibilities for young people's empowerment. Crucially, these different forms of empowerment intersect to shape and reproduce relations of power and offer different (and sometimes competing) possibilities for health promotion.

Conceptualizing empowerment

Chapter Two detailed a number of existing conceptualizations and the uses of the term *empowerment*. The discussion not only exemplifies the increasing popularity of empowerment in a range of contexts, but also points to a number of theoretical tensions and inconsistencies in use. As previously described, definitions of empowerment vary considerably in the emphasis placed on individual or collective approaches, and empowerment as a process and/or outcome (Rissel 1994, Rodwell 1996, Tones and Tilford 2001, Laverack 2009, Wiggins 2011). Much of the mainstream health promotion literature draws a distinction between psychological or individual empowerment (primarily drawing on theories from social psychology) and community or collective empowerment (drawing on theories from community development and specifically, Freire's [1996] notion of *conscientização* or critical consciousness raising).

Within this body of literature, empowerment is frequently presented as a bottom-up process whereby individuals and groups identify their own concerns and the means to address these concerns (Labonte 1993, Laverack 2009). This understanding of the concept captures the idea that empowerment is developed and gained by people themselves rather than granted or given by others (Tones 1998a and b, Williams and Labonte 2007, Laverack 2009), the latter implicitly suggesting the imposition of *power over* by those more powerful (Labonte 1989, 1993, Gomm 1993).

Empowerment has been further described as a continuum from individual to collective action (Labonte 1993, Laverack 2007, 2009) whereby increases in self-esteem and self-efficacy (individual empowerment) are widely considered as creating possibilities for collective consciousness raising and critical action (community empowerment). Critical action is then, somewhat unproblematically, viewed as capable of triggering changes in the social conditions negatively affecting health (Delp, Brown and Domenzain 2005, Wiggins 2011). This rather linear conceptualization highlights how processes of empowerment, in terms of building an individual's self-esteem and self-efficacy, may in themselves be seen as health promoting (Tones 1998a and b, Tones and Tilford 2001) but are also necessary prerequisites for the next 'stage' of empowerment and more collective responses (*ibid.*). It is the combination of these individual and collective processes that is said to prompt changes in the social context or, more often, the health status of individuals and groups (Laverack 2009, Wiggins 2011).

For example, Scriven and Stiddard's (2003) analysis of empowerment has illustrated how increases to young people's personal competencies through the development of health-related knowledge and skills can be instrumental in bringing about changes in the school environment, including the introduction of healthy food and increasing opportunities to engage in physical activity. Similarly, Wight and Dixon (2004, p. 5) described how modifying individual cognitions by increases in confidence and self-efficacy can help young people better negotiate sexual encounters.

These discussions, however, offer a rather unidirectional understanding of empowerment and present a somewhat preidentified endpoint or a set of particularly desired empowered outcomes, such as increasing young people's engagement in physical activity or negotiating condom use with partners. What this literature has failed to address, however, are the ways in which processes of empowerment may also result in more variable and indeterminate consequences or outcomes that may not be deemed health promoting by official perspectives. These *unintended* outcomes of processes of empowerment may, in turn, shape subsequent responses to these unintended outcomes by both young people and adults, suggesting a far more complex relationship between processes and outcomes of empowerment than hitherto articulated in the literature.

For instance, an increasing body of literature has shown how increases in young people's self-esteem can contribute to the decision to act against official health advice as an expression of autonomy and resistance to health promotion (West and Sweeting 1997, McGee and Williams 2000, Turner and Gordon 2004, Katainen 2006). The tendency to assume that processes of empowerment will result in actions that are in line with officially defined positive health practices and outcomes ignores the different priorities some young people may have in relation to their health and alternative ways to promote it (Percy-Smith 2007, Willis *et al.* 2008, Spencer 2008, 2013b).

There is also little recognition in the current literature of the ways in which processes of empowerment are themselves shaped and determined by context. In the study described here, young people's positive self-belief (as a possible indicator of more individualized forms of empowerment) was found to be closely linked to young people's social position (cf. Shoveller *et al.* 2004). Consequently, understanding what influences young people's discussions of a positive self-belief, for example, is important because any changes to these (social) factors may well impact (positively or negatively) on processes of empowerment.

In some cases, the possibility that outcomes from processes of empowerment may inadvertently contribute to the reproduction of some of the social conditions that appeared to negatively influence young people's health warrants further analysis. Young people's resistance to dominant perspectives through, for example, questioning adult authority, often had the effect of confirming the opinion that young people were disruptive, thereby strengthening the very authority young people sought to challenge (see Chapter Six).

Examples such as these illustrate some of the more complex and less determinate ways processes and outcomes of empowerment can result in the reinforcement of the status quo rather than bringing about the forms of social change suggested in much of the current literature.

As I have argued throughout this book, a significant omission in many existing discussions on empowerment has been a full-fledged engagement with the workings of power. The multiple ways in which power has been theorized hold different possibilities for understanding related concepts of empowerment (see Chapter Three). Undertheorized notions of power in much of the literature on empowerment have a tendency to oversimplify the relationship between empowerment and health. By unproblematically linking increases in individual self-esteem and self-efficacy with positive health outcomes, the current literature downplays the diverse ways in which power shapes the social structures and contexts in which health is enacted and experienced. Goldenberg *et al.* (2008), for example, exposed some of the broader social factors (age, gender and income) impacting on young people's sexual health. These wider factors were seen to shape the particular vulnerabilities young people experienced (and their opportunities to act) as a consequence of their location within a specific social context (see also Shoveller *et al.* 2004, 2010).

Toward a conceptual framework for understanding empowerment

Informed by Lukes's (2005) tripartite perspective of power, and drawing on young people's own narratives, I now take forward these concerns through the development of a new conceptual framework for understanding empowerment (see Figure 1). This new framework helps to better understand the complex relationship between power and empowerment as they affect young people's health. This form of analysis brings to the fore some of the tensions within existing theorizations of empowerment but also offers the opportunity to examine the constructive possibilities for social change in line with young people's own perspectives on health.

Fundamental to the development of this new conceptual framework for understanding empowerment is the acknowledgement of at least two different understandings of young people's health. The first, more dominant, perspective is premised on the normative frames of reference that guide current official health discourses. Analysis of policy and health-related literature reveals the predominance of concepts of risk, with particular attention given to negative health outcomes and 'risky' health-related practices. These dominant perspectives provide varying but often very limited understandings of how contextual and structural features affect health perspectives, practices and outcomes.

However, in this study and in the wider literature on young people's health, participants' own accounts of health often emphasized how their

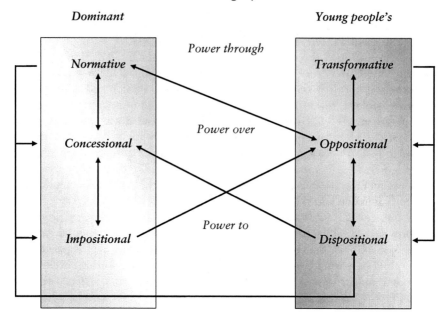

Figure 1 A Conceptual Framework for Empowerment

immediate environment and their relationships with significant others affected their health (cf. Shoveller *et al.* 2004). Young people's accounts also offered alternative, more positive discourses about health with potentially counter-hegemonic tendencies. By examining these alternative perspectives on health alongside more mainstream perspectives, some of the limitations of existing conceptualizations of empowerment can be revealed.

The proposed framework for empowerment is organized around these two understandings of health (the dominant and alternative) and draws in particular on Lukes's three dimensions of power: *power to, power over* and *power through*. The framework identifies six different, but coexisting forms of empowerment: *impositional, dispositional, concessional, oppositional, normative and transformative* (see Table 2). These new forms of empowerment intersect with one another (see Figure 1) and differentially, and sometimes inconsistently, shape possibilities for, and limitations of, empowerment for health.

Power to . . . Impositional and dispositional forms of empowerment

As described in Part One of this book, much of the existing literature on young people's health has a tendency to support a *power to* conceptualization

Table 2 Conceptual Framework for Understanding Empowerment

	Underpinning concepts of power and emerging forms of empowerment		
	Power to . . . the capacity or agency to act	*Power over . . .* exert control over others	*Power through . . .* dominant knowledge systems and accepted social truths
Dominant/ 'official' framings of health	*Impositional empowerment* – refers to the imposition of power, which reflects dominant systems of meaning. This top-down form of empowerment seeks to bring into effect normative ideas about what it means to be healthy.	*Concessional empowerment* – refers to accommodation and compromise being reached within formal systems of enacting change and within a prescribed range of predefined options.	*Normative empowerment* – refers to the reproduction of dominant knowledge systems. Resistance to normative assumptions serves to strengthen dominant relations of power.
Young people's 'alternative' framings of health	*Dispositional empowerment* – refers to young people's inclination to act within a given social context – giving way to 'episodic' moments of power.	*Oppositional empowerment* – refers to young people's opposing agendas and concerns, including their counterdiscourses and practices.	*Transformative empowerment* – refers to shifts in power through subverting dominant systems of meaning that give rise to social change.

First published by Sage Publishing Limited.

of individual empowerment by calling for the development of young people's self-esteem, confidence and motivation to increase personal control and enact 'healthy' decision making (see for example, Tisdall and Davis 2004, Pearson 2006, Morton and Montgomery 2011). Drawing heavily on normative and developmental frames of reference from within social psychology, this individualistic approach is reflected in recent official health discourses that stress the importance of increasing young people's knowledge and personal skills to reduce or stop their engagement in health-related practices that might be considered risky or harmful to health (see Australian Government 2010, Department of Health [DH] 2010b). Implicit within these accounts is the idea that many young people are deficient in certain skills and (psychological) attributes arising from their perceived lack of maturity. This 'immaturity' positions young people as being largely incapable of making informed, positive and healthy decisions for themselves and can be seen in recent health discourses on young people and their health:

> Working with communities and schools to develop young people's confidence and self-esteem. Empowering them to take better decisions when young, so that they enjoy greater health and well-being through life. . . . So that young people see drug use and binge-drinking not as a sign of being adult, but as evidence of their immaturity. (Lansley 2010, Speech to the UK Faculty of Public Health)

These individualized and imposed understandings of the concept thus constitute what might be described as an *impositional* form of empowerment. In contrast to the bottom-up strategies for empowerment discussed in much of the literature (see Laverack 2007, 2009); this impositional form is more prescriptive and organized around the development of young people's individual capacity and *power to* enact informed healthy decisions in line with official health perspectives.

Evidence of this impositional form of empowerment was seen frequently in this study. In the school environment, display boards, tutor time and some lessons emphasized the importance of developing self-esteem and confidence as key prerequisites for young people's health and well-being. Similarly, the accounts given by professionals, and some young people themselves, seemed to stress the importance of these more individualized uses of empowerment. The descriptions given by adults working with young people drew particular attention to young people's 'problematic' behaviours and the potential negative impact these had on their health. In particular, some adults stressed the value of increasing young people's self-esteem and confidence to enable them to resist 'peer pressure' and thereby promote their health in line with official health discourses.

> I think there's an awful amount of peer pressure to do things, they often feel pushed into situations and they don't have the confidence to protect themselves. (School Welfare Officer)

Similar examples were evident in young people's discussions of their home lives. As evidenced in Chapter Six, young people described how their parents were concerned about the effects of peer pressure and young people's potential engagement in risky health practices when out with friends, such as drinking alcohol or having sex. This parental concern was described by young people as limiting their opportunities to be with friends as parents often set clear boundaries about when, and with whom, young people could go out.

This impositional understanding of empowerment, however, is conceptually problematic when examining its links to young people's health. First, as illustrated, this form of empowerment is based on the imposition of dominant ideas of what it means to be healthy and thus undermines the notion that empowerment is something developed and gained by (young) people themselves (Williams and Labonte 2007, Laverack 2009, Wiggins 2011). Not only does such a top-down form of empowerment assume that young people can be empowered by others, but crucially this understanding of the concept fails to question whether young people themselves see such a form of empowerment as being an effective way to promote their health.

Second, impositional empowerment assumes that young people will be empowered through increases to their individual self-esteem and confidence. This downplays the effects of the structures and ideologies that shape (and frequently limit) the possibilities for (young people's) empowerment (Williams and Labonte 2007, Shoveller *et al.* 2010). Moreover, in this study, whilst young people occasionally referred to notions of confidence and self-esteem in their discussions of health, their accounts drew greater attention to the relational aspects of developing a 'positive belief in the self'. Young people's accounts of their positive self-belief were closely tied to ideas of *knowing I can do something*, *looking good*, and *talking to others* (Chapter Five). These aspects of young people's positive self-belief were rarely discussed in terms of individualized and decontextualized processes of personal development but more often reflected the importance young people gave to their social position as a factor influencing how they felt about themselves (cf. Room and Sato 2002) and crucially, how young people's self-belief was shaped by context in general, and gendered power relations in particular.

Melissa: For example, like with boys and I was liking one of them, if I look good, like confidence to go over to them and just start chatting to them (Silver group).

Researcher: What things help you believe in yourself?
Charlotte: Well the people around me telling me I can do something (Gold group).

Third, by suggesting the *need* to empower young people, impositional forms of empowerment appear to adopt a zero-sum perspective of power in which young people are constructed as being relatively powerless to act – a position young people in this study often sought to challenge. Such an approach runs counter to the more positive, animated and 'ludic' ways young people described their health in terms of being happy and having fun. By drawing attention to deficits and negative behaviours, this form of empowerment may actually reinforce the same negative discourses young people saw as adversely affecting their health and shows how processes of empowerment may also carry unintended (and negative) outcomes. As the discussion later illustrates, these unintended consequences or outcomes of empowerment shape subsequent responses by young people and adults and thus influence further possibilities for, and limits to, social change.

Fourth, and finally, impositional forms of empowerment downplay evidence of young people's *power to* act according to their own understandings of health, which (in this study at least) were often different from the more top-down, imposed meanings found in official health discourses. Although young people were aware of, and at times played back, these dominant perspectives, they also framed their own health in more positive ways. These alternative perspectives on health provide examples of young people's *power to* define and act in line with their own understandings of health – drawing attention to a second form of empowerment based on a *power to* conceptualization.

In contrast to the deficit model that characterizes impositional forms of empowerment, young people usually demonstrated their knowledge of official health perspectives and alternatively provided a more nuanced appreciation of how their health was both constrained and facilitated by contextual factors, such as the school environment. These contextual factors provided different opportunities for young people to act and promote their health according to their own frames of reference. For instance, young people were often seen to create their own and innovative ways to enjoy themselves by defining what was seen as being 'fun' within the classroom or when out with friends.

These moments of fun provided evidence of young people's *power to* act according to their own perspectives on health but also of how their opportunity to do so was often determined (and limited) by the various ways in which adults (re)asserted their authority – for example, by preventing young people from 'hanging around' in parks or by enforcing school rules. Both these actions served to limit the collective opportunities young people felt they had to enact the more positive and pleasurable aspects of their health.

Gina: They're keeping young people off the streets so people don't get irritated, not for our health . . . the government themselves don't really make a big deal out of how to make young people happy, they do it of more how to get them off the streets, they don't think about the happiness, just how to get rid of us (Gold group).

Similarly, some young people, particularly those from the Bronze group, thought that opportunities to demonstrate their *power to* act were limited by the ways in which the school had positioned them as being largely incapable of making important decisions about their lives. In contrast, in their descriptions of life at home, these same young people offered examples of their abilities to take on a number of responsibilities as they (independently) managed family health problems or provided care for younger siblings.

Here, examples of young people's propensity or inclination to act can be seen as a second or *dispositional* form of empowerment, highlighting the ways in which their *power to* act was determined (and often limited) by the broader social context and, in particular, those around them. Crucially, this latter form of empowerment captures the important *social* aspects of young people's health that were seen to create some possibilities for empowerment in line with young people's own perspectives and experiences.

Whilst both dispositional and impositional forms of empowerment are informed by a *power to* conceptualization of power, these two understandings of empowerment are conceptually distinct as the former does not imply young people's lack of capacity to act but instead stresses how an inclination to act is shaped by social context. By drawing attention to the importance of context in shaping young people's possibilities for empowerment, this second understanding of the concept helps better explain why young people may appear to act inconsistently in different situations and contexts.

Power over . . . Concessional and oppositional forms of empowerment

In the literature on young people's health there are numerous examples of young people's involvement in shaping health-related agendas and more participatory efforts to elicit young people's perspectives on health concerns (Rindner 2002, Cavet and Sloper 2004, Ataöv and Haider 2006, Percy-Smith 2007, Percy-Smith and Thomas 2010). In line with recent participation agendas emanating from the United Nations Convention on the Rights of the Child (UNCRC) (UN Assembly 1989, Department for Children, Schools and Families [DCSF] 2007, DH 2004a, Skidmore, Bound and Lownsbrough 2006), these perspectives stress the importance of developing partnership approaches to the promotion of young people's health. As described by the DCSF (2007, p. 23), 'Successful provision includes young people in its design and development, its running and its decision-making processes. This gives them a sense of empowerment'.

Whilst these participatory approaches appear to align with a more bottom-up strategy informed by young people's own concerns, these types of decision-making processes are often located within a predefined range of options based on adult-led priorities (cf. Wilson 2009, Pinkey 2011). This approach to young people's health might therefore be described as a *concessional* form of empowerment. Whilst concessional forms of empowerment may accommodate young people's views, they rely largely on agreement being reached within adult-framed and controlled systems of change. Changes to social context may take place, but these are often tokenistic concessions made to sustain an impression of young people having *power over* changes to their own lives.

Evidence of concessional forms of empowerment was also seen frequently in this study. Within the school environment, young people's participation and *power over* setting health-related priorities was actively encouraged through various formalized committees such as the school council and school parliament. Teachers and some young people viewed these fora positively as giving young people the opportunity to express their opinions and influence matters of concern to them.

Despite some evidence of support for these committees, criticisms were made by many young people regarding the ability of such mechanisms to take their concerns seriously. Fora such as the school council were frequently described as 'serving the interests of the school' rather than responding to the concerns of young people themselves, such as changes to school food or improvements in the condition of the school toilets. Of particular concern to young people were the ways in which they felt the school council merely created an illusion of their having *power over,* through concessionary and tokenistic actions.

> *Ian:*   I don't want to sound like really sceptic, but it's just like a cover, they just wanna seem they're like taking the views of the pupils into account when they're actually just doing what they want (Gold group).

Tokenism with regards to participation is highlighted in findings of other research, particularly with respect to the marginalization of young people's perspectives (Alderson 2000, Johnny 2006, Wilson 2009). These broader discussions, and evidence from this study, highlight young people's awareness of the assumed participatory intentions of concessional forms of empowerment and the exclusionary mechanisms that may operate within them. In this study, young people's accounts signalled their resistance to the systems and structures they thought failed to take seriously young people's own perspectives.

This reported failure to take young people's perspectives seriously – a finding widely echoed elsewhere in the literature (Cavet and Sloper 2004, Boylan and Ing 2005, Warwick *et al.* 2005, Wilson 2009) – was not only thought to limit opportunities to influence the shaping of school priorities but was also closely linked to the expression of views and ideas that contrasted with received adult opinion. Specifically, when offering a different opinion from that of teachers and other adults, young people described the negative reactions they received, including being sent out of class or being 'grounded' by parents.

> *Rob:*   If they say what is your opinion on something, and then you say something they don't want to hear, you can get told off for it because it's not what they want to hear.
>
> *Researcher:*   So when they ask you for your opinion what do you think they expect?
>
> *Rob:*   Exactly, I think they just expect along the lines what they wanna hear . . . they don't like your opinion. They're sort of telling you what they're supposed to tell you, but it's not always how it is in real life (Gold group).

Consequently, although concessional forms of empowerment may offer opportunities for young people to express opinions within the school, these opportunities were thought to be open only when young people's views aligned with the opinion of teachers and other adults. Validation of young people's perspectives as being either 'right' or 'wrong' exemplified how adults often retained *power over* which (and whose) views were deemed permissible to express within any given context. Marginalizing young people's views in such a way limited the opportunities young people had to exercise their own *power over* decision-making and effectively excluded their opinions from reaching (and influencing) mainstream discussion.

For example, when questioning the perceived fairness of school or parental rules or sanctions, young people described how their attempts to put forward their views were frequently interpreted as being disruptive and disrespectful. Although on some occasions adults would listen to their perspectives (although did not always act on them), the dismissal of young people's opinions more often served to undermine the integrity of young people's perspectives as a valued form of knowing. By framing young people's opinions as 'wrong', dominant framings reduced young people's perspectives to a position of invalidity and not to be trusted. Examining young people's responses to these processes of invalidation, however, highlighted an alternative and fourth understanding of empowerment based on a *power over* conceptualization.

Crucially, young people's challenges to adult perspectives provided evidence of a form of critical consciousness that might prefigure more collective forms of empowerment. In this study, young people were often seen to question or make fun of the perspectives of teachers in their discussions with friends. Similarly, on a number of occasions within the school, young people questioned adult opinion by 'answering back'. These examples of young people's resistance to dominant perspectives may be seen as an *oppositional* form of empowerment. This oppositional empowerment engages with and represents critical issues for young people as defined by them and seeks to promote young people's own agendas and concerns, including their counter-discourses and practices.

Of most concern to young people were the various (negative) judgements made about them, which they thought signalled a widespread lack of trust and respect for young people generally. These misrepresentations were not only reported to impact negatively on young people's health but often sparked resistance. Whilst on some (rare) occasions, young people's 'resistance' (as a form of oppositional empowerment) actually subverted the normal order of the school, these challenges to dominant systems of meaning were largely viewed by adults as being disruptive and often resulted in efforts to reinforce school or parental rules.

In line with a body of literature examining concepts of resistance within youth subcultures (Clarke *et al.* 1976, Jefferson 1976, Aggleton 1987, Raby 2002, 2005, 2010), this oppositional form of empowerment therefore had little effect on changing dominant systems of meaning and effectively *reinforced* dominant relations of power because, all too often, young people's oppositional actions were taken as evidence of their 'immature' and disruptive behaviour (this latter point is examined more closely in the subsequent discussion on *power through* forms of empowerment).

Because of this, we may properly see many oppositional forms of empowerment as instances of contestation (cf. Aggleton 1987). Whilst in some circumstances critical consciousness-raising might be considered the first step toward more collective empowerment, in this study young people's awareness of the *power over* them did not bring about major changes in the school environment and often had the *unintended* consequence of reinforcing existing relations of power. These unintended consequences of opposition provide further evidence of some of the more negative outcomes that can arise from empowerment. These unintended outcomes, in turn, shaped subsequent responses by adults as young people were often sanctioned for their 'disruptive' behaviour.

Awareness of the power others exercised over young people more often than not resulted in expressions of frustration and an unwillingness to act. This lack of action did not, however, signal a form of 'false consciousness' or the effects of young people's 'disempowerment'. Indeed, young people in this study were highly critical of the diverse ways in which power was exercised over them and demonstrated considerable insight into the ways in which their resistance contributed to, and strengthened, adult sanctions. Instead, young people's apparent lack of action signalled their frustration at the tendency of many adults to dismiss their ways of knowing and the limits to which young people could effectively challenge adult opinion. These limits often led young people to believe there was little point in trying to effect change. However, it was in young people's accounts of their abstaining (as a form of oppositional empowerment) that we can begin to see some constructive possibilities for changing dominant systems of power.

Although relatively rare in this study, there were times when young people appeared to simply comply with the directions of adults for one of two key reasons. First, young people were aware of the dangers of reinforcing the view that they were troublesome by challenging adult opinion. Second, young people believed that dominant negative images of young people were so far removed from the reality of their own lives that they often described how they simply could not be 'bothered' to engage with these perspectives and frequently complied with the directions of adults as a consequence.

Simon: You just think why bother, they're not gunna listen so why bother saying anything to try and change anything (Gold group).

Sarah: It makes you feel why bother? They're gunna think that no matter what you do, so why bother trying to change that? (Gold group).

Evidence of young people's apparent compliance with adult authority, however, did not signal their acquiescence or agreement but illustrated the extent to which they strongly disagreed with the idea that young people were inherently bad. Displaying what seemed to be a form of passivity was a powerful way in which young people were able to challenge dominant problematizing discourses by appearing to simply accept and conform to the directions of adults. This more subtle form of what I term here 'resistance through inaction' can be seen in the following account:

Rob: I've been pulled over a few times . . . we walking back to my mate's house . . . and the police they just stopped us. . . . They've asked to search our bag and 'cos obviously they're police you've just gotta do what they say otherwise you'll get done, it's like, they just stereotype you, teenagers always get accused of doing something and we just gotta do what they say (Gold group).

Examples of this kind illustrate that what might on first impression appear to be inconsistencies in young people's accounts and actions; young people's displays of resistance *and* apparent 'abstention' can be better understood as two related strategies of opposition to dominant perspectives but with differing outcomes and effects.

Power through . . . Normative and transformative forms of empowerment

Lukes's third dimension of power is explicitly ideological in nature and draws attention to the processes of social and cultural reproduction that legitimize dominant frameworks of understanding as being part of the natural order of society. Critical social theory and more recent poststructuralist understandings of power have examined these processes of social and cultural reproduction in detail and have sought to illustrate the potential ways young people's resistance to dominant discourses may shift relations of power. Drawing on Gramsci's (1971) concept of hegemony, for example, early youth subcultural studies examined young people's resistant and counter-hegemonic practices, with a particular focus on the reproduction of class and other inequalities (Clarke *et al.* 1976, Jefferson 1976, Willis 1977, Aggleton 1987). More recent work, often informed by Foucauldian perspectives on power (Foucault 1980), has similarly examined the potential for young people's resistance to dominant (gender) discourses to shift power relations (Allen 2003a and b, Renold 2004, Youdell 2005, Juelskjær 2008, Raby 2010, Doull and Sethna 2011).

In this study, the consequences of *power through* frameworks of understanding were closely tied to the social category of age and, in particular, the reproduction of widespread assumptions that link 'adolescence' to a developmental period and time of risk. These dominant perspectives about adolescence were frequently replayed in both the accounts of adults and those of some young people in this study. Teachers and other professionals working with young people often made reference to the links between youth, immaturity and risk and understood this as part of the normal 'storm and stress' of adolescent development (Hall 1904).

> I think it's just the age they're at, young people of that age, I think they're succeeding within their peer group, because they're seen as the one that will take risks, the one that's game for anything. But if they dared to stop and think about it . . . but I guess it's just about growing up isn't it? (Social and Emotional Aspects of Learning coordinator)

Young people themselves were also seen to take up and reproduce these perspectives. Drawing on (negative) images of young people in the media, participants across all groups appeared to adhere to notions of the risky young Other (Hollingworth and Williams 2009, Spencer 2013c). At times, some young people, particularly those in the Bronze and Silver groups, questioned their abilities to achieve in both academic and nonacademic activities. Other young people appeared to devalue their nonadult status and aspired to a future more competent self through the suggestion that they were too young to influence matters of importance until they themselves were adults.

Researcher: Do you feel you can influence things in your life?
Claire: I don't because I'm a child (Gold group).

The reproduction of these dominant perspectives also revealed a gendered dimension. Young men in the study were more often linked to problematizing discourses than young women. Specifically, in Chapter Five young men described how their appearance often attracted (negative) attention and how their behaviour was seen as being disruptive or 'antisocial' by teachers and members of the public. These assumptions about young men's behaviour were further linked to their stage of (im)maturity and biological development.

Lisa: I think it's just boys, like they don't mature to like when they're 18.
Researcher: So you think there's a difference between the boys and girls?
Lisa: Yeah, the boys the same age are just so immature compared to girls. . . . Boys seriously don't mature . . . but their brain, it's actually a true statement though isn't it that their brain is a year below us, like their brain isn't properly developed until they're 18 (Gold group).

Young people's own use of these dominant perspectives was particularly pronounced when they were attempting to explain social differences between themselves, other young people and adults. These illustrations exemplified how *generation* not only defined and shaped the everyday lives and experiences of young people (Mannheim 1952, Alanen and Mayall 2001, Jupp 2007), but also divided participants from other young people. The different ways young people reproduced these perspectives highlighted the pervasive ways *power through* dominant discourses limited the opportunities for young people to recognize themselves as sharing a 'common social location' (Mannheim 1952), creating significant barriers for the possibilities of realizing collective empowerment. Furthermore, any recognition of young people occupying a 'common social location' rather paradoxically would seem to require young people to identify themselves as being young – thereby potentially aligning themselves with the normative assumptions they also used to describe other young people.

Of significance to the reproduction of these perspectives was the contribution of health promotion. Through its focus on risks to health, whilst emphasizing the need to build young people's self-esteem, health promotion initiatives were heavily criticized by young people for portraying a largely negative picture of young people and their health based on assumptions about their (im)maturity and engagement in risky health behaviours. This negative approach not only marginalized the more positive ways young people described their health (thereby downplaying the promotion of health according to young people's own frames of reference) but also supported the suggestion that immaturity and risk are specific to those of a particular (younger) age.

Despite evidence of assimilation, more often than not young people identified these discourses and their effects as discriminatory and a form of 'ageism'. Indeed, young people frequently described the unfair treatment they experienced as a consequence of their nonadult status (cf. Morrow 2000, 2001, Mason and Fallon 2001, Tucker 2003, Mannion 2007) and, specifically, the negative effects that being seen as immature and troublesome had on their health.

Lucy:	I don't think that adults or people in society realize that when they put this image of teenagers all being yobs that they're actually affecting the teenagers. I know that we just live with it as a way of life, the fact that people expect us to be bad and horrible. We shouldn't have to feel like that.
Researcher:	When you say 'you feel it', how does it make you feel?
Lucy:	It makes you unhappy, it makes you feel worthless, you're like why should I bother, if all they think of me is that. It does make you feel bad (Gold group).

Despite such criticisms, participants did not recognize themselves as sharing a common social location that may prefigure collective forms of empowerment. Instead, during discussions about their own health, many young people challenged ideas about their immaturity by suggesting they were quite knowledgeable about the risks associated with health behaviours such as smoking and drinking (cf. Skidmore and Hayter 2000, Denscombe 2001a and b, Stjerna, Lauritzen and Tillgren 2004, Baillie *et al.* 2005, Katainen 2006). Whilst these discussions may indicate something of the recent success of health education in schools in the UK (see DfES/DH 2005, Warwick *et al.* 2005), these accounts also demonstrated young people's criticisms of some of the widely held assumptions about young people, risk and health. Respondents often stressed their abilities to make their own decisions about their health. Indeed, examples of their dispositional empowerment provided evidence of young people's ability to act according to their own understandings of health. However, by acting against official health discourses (and the normative assumptions they make about age), young people in this study unwittingly reinforced the adult view that they were not responsible or mature enough to make positive decisions for themselves.

Evidence of young people's criticisms of these dominant perspectives points to a form of empowerment that seeks to challenge many of the normative assumptions linked to their nonadult status. However, outcomes of this form of empowerment were seen to be highly *reproductive* in that they strengthened and reproduced existing power relations. This form of empowerment may therefore be described as *normative*. Normative empowerment draws attention to the ways in which *power through* dominant frameworks of knowledge come to define and legitimate currently accepted social 'truths'. Whilst these truths were often contested by young people in both their narratives and practices, these challenges ultimately served to reinforce and reproduce dominant frameworks of understanding and relations of power.

Once again, examples of normative empowerment were frequently seen in this study. Young people often criticized the school's cohort system, which not only seemed to reflect wider social norms about young people's differing developmental capabilities (cf. Darbyshire, MacDougall and Schiller 2005, Allen 2007, Jupp 2007) but also reflected the idea that young people displaying 'challenging behaviour' required specific treatment. Young people themselves, however, perceived these structuring processes as evidence of the school's preferential treatment of some young people. For some young people, particularly those from the Bronze group, this differential treatment of various groups of young people was thought to limit their options in later life. Whilst teachers often justified this approach as 'protecting' young people's 'best interests', members of the Bronze group described how assumptions made about their abilities and behaviour ultimately 'fixed' them in a lower social position.

A further example drawn from observational work highlighted how assumptions about age downplayed evidence of dominant gender power relations. During a science lesson Carl (a member of the Gold group) challenged the accuracy of information presented by the (female) teacher. This challenge was quickly dismissed, and Carl was sent out of the lesson for causing a 'disruption'. In a subsequent science lesson, it was confirmed by the head of science that Carl's challenge was indeed correct. Despite this public admission, the teacher concerned refused to concede the point and appeared to avoid the topic despite Carl's insistence that she simply confirm that he had been right and she was wrong. The teacher's final comment was to suggest that Carl's challenge was typical of 'boys being boys'.

These examples of young people's normative empowerment offer an understanding of how the operation of *power through* the social category of age not only continued to position young people as inferior but also worked alongside other forms of social organization such as those linked to social class and gender (cf. Mason and Fallon 2001). Crucially, young people's age appeared to operate as a vehicle through which other forms of inequality were effectively 'explained away' to maintain and strengthen prevailing regimes of power.

Importantly, young people did at times demonstrate an awareness of the reproductive outcomes of normative empowerment. For example, Carl later described how his labelling as disruptive by his science teacher made any further challenges to this or other teachers' knowledge problematic. Meanwhile, the girls in the Bronze group described how developing aspirations for themselves in terms of their future career pathways (such as wanting to be hairdressers or chefs) confirmed the perspective that they lacked knowledge about the 'real' world and a full understanding about what such high aspirations might involve.

It was during young people's discussions of the reproductive effects of normative forms of empowerment that some constructive possibilities for challenging *power through* dominant frameworks of understanding emerged. In their accounts of how best to promote health (which usually focused on the positive aspects of their health), young people expressed a strong desire to change the widely held (negative) assumptions made about them. In particular, young people called on adults (including government and media) to promote a more positive perspective about young people through highlighting the contributions they made to society.

Dean: I think they need to focus more on the good sides, like what we do for the community, it's like we're equal as the next person, we're just the same, we're still members of society (Bronze group).

In their accounts, young people sought to create new or alternative discourses, rather than purely challenge existing discourses (cf. Ungar and Teram 2000). Specifically, a refocusing of dominant (negative) perspectives to offer a more positive image of young people was thought to be the most effective way to bring about the types of social change they believed necessary to promote their health. These discussions suggest a further understanding of empowerment based on a *power through* conceptualization. This form of empowerment can be understood as potentially *transformative* and indicates some constructive possibilities for changing prevailing power relations between young people and adults.

Although relatively rare in this study, possibilities for transforming dominant understandings of young people were observed in the more positive relationships some young people (most notably those in the Gold group) had developed with particular adults. These examples were characterized by young people as displaying a relationship based on a more reciprocal notion of respect. For young people in this study, respect was understood as a two-way exchange between adults and young people and, specifically, was based on adults taking seriously young people's perspectives as valid forms of knowing.

For example, participants described how some adults appeared to hold a more positive view of young people and felt they treated them, and their friends, with more respect as a consequence (see Chapter Seven). Crucially, young people reported the positive effects these experiences had on their health. In particular, being respected by adults made these young people feel included in discussions and valued as individuals, enabling them to better negotiate everyday interactions with adults.

However, although these examples of reciprocally respectful relationships between young people and adults may offer some constructive possibilities to shift power relations, this transformative form of empowerment presents a significant paradox for existing bottom-up theorizations of the concept. As young people's accounts acknowledged, the potential to realize transformative empowerment necessitated adults to legitimate young people's ways of knowing as valid forms of knowledge and praxis. For *transformative* empowerment to become possible therefore requires young people's *dispositional* empowerment to be accepted as evidence of their capabilities to act and shape their own lives in accordance with their own frames of reference. Similarly, *oppositional* forms of empowerment need to be viewed as collective attempts by young people to state their preferences and act according to their own perspectives (and not as evidence of young people's defiance and unruly behaviour).

Thus, the paradox for transformative forms of empowerment is that in the very act of legitimizing young people's perspectives as valid forms of knowing, power is ultimately exercised by those in a position of power (because they hold the potential to either legitimatize [or not] such perspectives as being valid). This operation of power again raises questions about the possibilities for understanding empowerment as a purely bottom-up approach as currently suggested in much of the health promotion literature.

Empowerment and its relationship to young people's health

I conclude this chapter by highlighting how these six newly developed ways of understanding empowerment may help to advance existing conceptualizations of the term and better explain the concept's relationship to health. By doing so, this final discussion addresses some of the key theoretical tensions identified in existing understandings of the concept. Specifically, the discussion highlights how differentiating between processes and outcomes of empowerment may be an unhelpful distinction to apply when examining the concept's relationship to health, and why understanding empowerment as a bottom-up approach may be also problematic.

This study's findings suggest that a more dynamic and generative understanding of empowerment than hitherto articulated may be necessary to account for the relationship between empowerment and young people's health. As depicted in Figure 1, the dynamic nature of the concept is evident through the multiple ways in which different forms of empowerment can shape and influence relations of power which, in turn, define the possible effects of that power. The generative features of the concept bring to the fore the diverse (and often competing) ways in which outcomes of empowerment may, in turn, shape subsequent responses by both young people and adults, creating both further possibilities for, and limitations of, young people's own capacity to act.

For example, evidence of young people's dispositional and oppositional empowerment pointed to the diverse ways in which participants acted in accordance with their own understandings of health. In their discussions, young people stressed their abilities to make decisions for themselves by drawing on the notion of choice. Young people's discussions of choice, however, also revealed the potential for participants to act in ways that ran contrary to adult judgement. By acting against dominant prescriptions in relation to health, young people's resistance inadvertently confirmed normative assumptions about their immaturity and propensity to engage in risky behaviour – thereby providing the very rationale to empower young people as articulated within dominant health discourses.

Teachers' efforts to promote the forms of empowerment consistent with dominant perspectives (identified here as impositional and concessional forms of empowerment), however, often triggered further resistance by young people, who sought to challenge these dominant ideas about themselves as being immature and disruptive. This resistance was perceived by teachers and other adults as confirming widely held perspectives on young people and thus, in turn, supporting normative forms of empowerment and the further reproduction of dominant power relations.

This illustration of how different forms of empowerment operate alongside but also against each other explains why differentiating between processes and outcomes, as much health promotion theory currently does, may be conceptually problematic. As findings from this study suggest, the (unintended) outcomes of one form of empowerment may create the need for another form of empowerment or limit the possibilities for other forms of empowerment to emerge. Such a relationship between processes and outcomes also highlights some of the generative potentials of the concept as different forms of empowerment trigger the possibility for other forms of empowerment to be realized. This more dynamic and generative conceptualization challenges the idea that empowerment is a relatively linear continuum and helps better explain why, in some circumstances, empowerment may or may not translate into the positive health outcomes as defined by official health discourse.

The outlined framework of empowerment can also help explain some of the apparent contradictions and anomalies in young people's accounts as different forms of empowerment were taken up in response to differing contexts (such as the school environment) and the forms of power operating within those contexts. Young people were seen to simultaneously resist and accommodate dominant perspectives in their own narratives and practices. These inconsistencies not only reproduced normative forms of empowerment (which in turn limited the degree to which other forms of empowerment became possible) but also revealed some of the weaknesses implicit in dominant discourses about young people.

For example, evidence of young people's 'resistance through inaction' revealed a powerful way in which young people challenged dominant problematizing discourses by appearing to conform to adult authority – thereby undermining the strength of the perspective that young people are inherently unruly and troublesome. Likewise, when questioned by teachers, some young people gave responses that appeared to suggest their compliance with adult-led perspectives in order to divert unwanted adult attention in the school context and show their apparent compliance with school rules. It is within these types of examples that the more transformative potentials of empowerment, based on young people's frames of reference, emerged.

In this study, young people underscored the value of a refocusing on a more positive conceptualization of young people and their health rather than the problems (in terms of potential health risks) to the possibility for a more transformative conceptualization of empowerment. Opportunities for realizing transformative forms of empowerment were, however, premised on the willingness of adults to at least temporarily bracket dominant (negative) images of young people and, by doing so, recognize the more positive contributions young people make. By foregrounding young people's ways of knowing, dominant (negative) discourses of young people may be challenged and replaced with more positive perspectives on young people and their health.

In this way, transformative forms of empowerment cannot be understood as purely bottom-up in their operation and effects because the realization of transformative forms of empowerment (at least in the school context) is itself contingent on adults challenging dominant perspectives and, specifically, legitimizing young people's systems of meaning as valid ways of knowing and acting. This understanding of the concept returns to one of the book's underpinning arguments, namely that understanding the theoretical and operational complexities of empowerment cannot be separated from an analysis of the workings and effects of *power* itself.

Conclusion

Informed by Lukes's tripartite perspective of power and drawing on two distinct understandings of health (the dominant and the alternative), in this chapter I have developed six different forms of empowerment (*impositional, dispositional, concessional, oppositional, normative, transformative*). These newly developed understandings of empowerment highlight a more dynamic and generative understanding of the concept than hitherto articulated in the literature. Such a dynamic and generative conceptualization advances the understanding of empowerment and helps to better explain the relationship between empowerment and young people's health.

9 Empowerment, health promotion and young people
Future directions

This close-focused examination of empowerment, health promotion and young people has sought to unpack some of the complexities underpinning concepts of empowerment and, in particular, to better explain the concept's relationship to, and relevance for, young people's health and health promotion. In this final chapter I consider some of the possible links between the six newly developed forms of empowerment and existing approaches to health promotion, along with some of the wider implications the presenting framework may hold for young people and health promotion more broadly. A number of future directions for policy and health promotion practice are identified, including a consideration of the potential relevance the new framework may hold for other young people from different social backgrounds, ethnicities and cultural contexts. I close with some final reflections on process. Here, I detail and reflect on some of the relative strengths, and challenges, of investigating concepts of empowerment and health with young people and how these insights may help to inform future enquiry on young people's health.

Empowerment and health promotion

Informed by different theorizations of power, this critical exploration of empowerment has troubled many of the existing meanings and uses of the concept within health promotion and specifically, in relation to young people's health. This form of analysis has helped to expose some previously unquestioned assumptions and thorny theoretical tensions within current uses and conceptions of empowerment. Based on findings from an empirical enquiry on empowerment, young people and health (Spencer 2011), a more dynamic and generative understanding of empowerment than has hitherto been present in the literature has been proposed.

Drawing on Lukes's (2005) tripartite perspective on power and examining two interrelated understandings of health (the dominant and the alternative), six conceptually distinct forms of empowerment have been identified (*impositional, dispositional, concessional, oppositional, normative, transformative*). The different ways in which these six forms of empowerment intersect to produce and reproduce relations of power helps to better explain some of the identified theoretical tensions within existing conceptualizations and, importantly, the possible relationship between empowerment and young people's health. These new conceptions of empowerment challenge existing understandings of the concept as a relatively linear continuum and further trouble the conceptual distinction made in the literature between processes and outcomes of empowerment.

The significance of these new forms of empowerment lies in the opportunities they may offer for health promotion theory and practice. By offering some alternative ways of understanding concepts of empowerment, this new conceptual framework lays the foundations for some different avenues and new forms of enquiry for investigating empowerment's relationship to health – not just with young people but perhaps too with other minority or marginalized groups, including younger children, adults from varying socioeconomic and educational backgrounds and with other groups of young people from differing sociocultural backgrounds and ethnicities.

Future directions for health promotion

As described, these six newly identified understandings of empowerment give rise to different understandings of the concept and offer some alternative (and potentially competing) 'sites' for health promotion. Much current health promotion is organized around what I have termed *impositional* and *concessional* forms of empowerment. Health promotion efforts to increase young people's self-esteem (and with a particular emphasis on reducing risky behaviours and promoting informed healthy decision making), for example, can be seen to reflect a more impositional approach. Meanwhile, health promotion efforts aligned with more concessional forms of empowerment have risen in popularity with the increasing emphasis on (young people's) participation and user involvement in health-related policy (see Department of Health [DH] 2010a and b). Thus, as part of the Healthy Schools' agenda in the United Kingdom (Department for Education and Skills/DH 2005), the widespread introduction of forums such as school councils and parliaments has attempted to operationalize ideas about the importance of young people's participation to promote their health.

Parallels can be drawn between these examples of impositional and concessional forms of empowerment and those more traditional behaviour change and educational approaches to health promotion that aim to develop an individual's knowledge, attitudes and beliefs in order to bring about changes to behaviour (see for example Ajzen and Fishbein 1980, Prochaska and DiClimente 1984, Tones and Tilford 2001). These latter approaches, however, pay rather limited attention to the crucial social and contextual influences on health and young people's health-related practices and experiences (cf. dispositional forms of empowerment). These impositional and concessional forms of empowerment therefore have a tendency to support and reinforce normative ideologies and practices that (according to the accounts of young people in this study) were part of the structures and ideologies negatively affecting their health. Health promotion initiatives of these kinds have demonstrated varying success in bringing about positive health outcomes in line with official health discourse (Webb and Sheeran 2008, Shepherd *et al.* 2010). The analysis offered here suggests a way of understanding this variability as much current health promotion policy and practice can be seen to sustain (rather than challenge) the very factors young people believed negatively affected their health.

Thus, the framework of empowerment developed here offers new ways of understanding the possible successes and challenges associated with other approaches to health promotion and provides further opportunities for the development of health promotion practice that takes young people's own understandings of health as their starting point. These 'alternative' opportunities for health promotion offer some new avenues of enquiry and evaluation to ascertain their potential effectiveness to bring about positive health, including their possible relevance for health promotion practice with other social groups.

Approaching health positively

In line with a now large body of literature that argues for taking young people's perspectives seriously (Mayall 2002, Alderson 2008, Christensen and James 2008, Qvortrup, Corsaro and Honig 2009), this book has argued for making young people's own understandings of *health* the starting point for health promotion and the importance of ensuring health promotion frameworks engage with young people's lived experiences.

By examining young people's accounts of 'feeling well', the analysis has revealed some of the different frames of reference young people draw upon in their understandings and experiences of health, which may well diverge from, and even challenge, dominant perspectives on health. Indeed, young people in this study drew frequent reference to the disjunction between what adults think about young people's health and the reality of their everyday lived experiences (cf. Percy-Smith 2006, 2007, Sixsmith *et al.* 2007, Willis *et al.* 2008). More specifically, young people called for future health promotion efforts to challenge the current negative and problem-based approach to young people's health – highlighting too the importance of the affective dimensions of young people's health (in terms of being happy and having fun).

Although not downplaying the challenges many young people face, current problematization of young people's health within official health promotion policies and discourses can be seen to work against the promotion of health as defined by young people themselves. In this study, young people underscored the particular value of bringing the more positive aspects of their lives to the fore rather than focusing attention on their assumed deficits or risk behaviours. These more positive and affirming understandings of health suggest the potential relevance of developing and extending more 'asset-based' approaches in health promotion with young people (Morgan and Ziglio 2007).

In line with these perspectives, future health-related policy and research might therefore question the value of topic-based approaches to young people's health that have a tendency to sustain a more negative focus on reducing risky behaviours such as binge-drinking, unsafe sex or illicit drug use. A refocusing on the positive would signal the potential to shift dominant individualized risk-reduction approaches to health in line with more transformative forms of empowerment that encapsulate the importance of reframing young people, and their health, in more positive ways. As the dynamic framework of empowerment put forward suggests, this reframing would then facilitate further opportunities for empowerment and continue generating such possibilities.

Valuing young people's contributions

Bringing young people's more positive expressions of health to the fore underscores the importance of ensuring greater acknowledgement of young people's efforts and achievements in all aspects of their lives. Doing well was seen to be an important contributor to young people's experiences of health and was particularly valued when coupled with positive recognition by others and, in particular, from adults. Although the school as an institution has been shown to reproduce inequities and power imbalances (see also Allen 2007, 2008, Jupp 2007), more could be done to acknowledge and value the contributions and achievements of *all* young people. Schools, in particular, could play an instrumental role in challenging negative community and societal views of young people by taking responsibility to emphasize young people's achievements and contributions. Sending positive examples of young people's schoolwork and social activities to the local press, or through feedback to parents and school governors, might help rebalance some of the negativity typically associated with young people.

More generally, and at a societal level, governments (both local and national), in collaboration with the media, have a pivotal role to play in laying the foundations for more transformative forms of empowerment by promoting more positive representations of young people. In particular, underscoring young people's abilities and capabilities rather than assumed deficits, through highlighting the contributions young people can and do make to the lives of others and society more generally would signify an important mark of respect for young people and their contributions.

Moving beyond official health priorities

Health promotion and public health more broadly need to continue to work toward challenging the structural and contextual features that (negatively) affect young people's health. Specifically, addressing young people's concerns that move beyond official health priorities may include increasing the provision and access to a range of affordable *and* meaningful activities and places to go for young people. Increasing opportunities to have fun, without this being reframed as negative or unruly behaviour, would mark an important step towards developing activities in line with young people's ways of seeing and promoting their health.

Increasing the availability of affordable activities for young people requires local and national governments to work *with* young people to identify desired activities that they feel better support their health. Identifying such activities should offer real opportunities for young people themselves to define and shape the type and range of activities available. In particular, young people's ownership over the activities they see as best supporting their health might include measures to increase the availability of safe, well-lit open spaces for young people – spaces respected by adults as being occupied by young people and free from (adult) surveillance. Extending activities that might help young people and adults come together in more power-sharing ways through, for example, enabling young people to access sports facilities or teams that are typically the preserve of adults may help support the development of the more reciprocal notions of respect young people described as being particularly important to the promotion of their health.

Identifying young people's health-related concerns

Identifying and acknowledging young people's health-related concerns as valid priorities for policy development, research and health promotion practice is an important step towards developing new forms of health promotion theory in line with young people's perspectives. Action at a number of levels is needed to systematically and sensitively ascertain the views and perspectives of young people from a range of social backgrounds. Far from being a tokenistic gesture, processes of accessing young people's perspectives need to move beyond concessional forms of empowerment and should be followed through with actions that put their suggestions into place. Taking young people's ideas on as a priority would mark an important step to valuing their perspectives, supporting opportunities to shift dominant understandings and accepting their ways of knowing as being valid.

Similarly, research on young people's health might usefully consider the value of starting from a more positive perspective on health and evaluating the potential effectiveness this more positive approach might have on achieving health equity and equality. This might include underscoring the social category of age as an important unit of analysis, alongside the more theorized and investigated dimensions of gender, social class and ethnicity. This could be approached in two ways: first, through an examination of the specific features and impacts of 'being young' on young people's health, and second, as a way of understanding how young people's experiences may be shaped and defined by the social category of 'age' itself.

Crucially, future research with a focus on the concept of empowerment should be more sensitive to the workings of power that shape the possibilities for, and limitations of, empowerment. In doing so, empowerment-based research should be critical of the underlying assumptions and potential effectiveness of the term *empowerment* and how it might link to (young people's) health or indeed align with more traditional approaches to health promotion, such as behaviour change strategies. This more critical approach will help to further the conceptual development (and consider the empirical evidence for) some of the different forms of empowerment developed in this book. In particular, future research might usefully examine how empowerment may operate in more dynamic and generative (rather than linear) ways, which may help to further understanding about the concept's relationship to health – for example, by examining more fully the social factors influencing the possibilities for forms of dispositional empowerment and how these social aspects may contribute to health.

Finally, research with young people should utilize methods shown to be most effective and acceptable to young people but should also display sensitivity to the context(s) in which data are collected and used (Hill 2006). In particular, researchers should question how research designs and forms of questioning might inadvertently contribute to dominant constructions of young people's health in more negative terms, or how they position young people within research (i.e., passive or active; troubled or risky). Identifying the methodologies and methods that best enable young people to articulate and share their realities is central to examining concepts of health and empowerment as they are experienced and understood by young people themselves.

Closing comments

In recent times, concepts of empowerment have been drawn upon in response to the widespread global attention on (and concern for) young people's health. Despite its popularity, the concept of empowerment has been applied rather critically to young people's health, often without a full-fledged engagement with the underpinning workings of power. Informed by concepts of power, this book has thus troubled some of the existing meanings and uses of empowerment as they relate to young people and health. This critical approach has enabled the development of a new conceptual framework of empowerment – crucially informed by young people's own frames of reference on health and underpinned by recent theorizations of power.

The close-focused study of empowerment, young people and health on which this newly developed framework for understanding empowerment is based was, however, conducted in just one locality in central England and thus, does not purport to capture the potentially diverse range of experiences and meanings given to health and empowerment by all young people. Although this investigation has offered important insights into the different factors young people see as important for their health, these findings may merely reflect the structures and discourses operating in that particular context (Jupp 2007). In light of these concerns, I now close by offering some reflections on some of the likely limits to this new framework for understanding empowerment. This short account aims to further illuminate some of the complexities encountered in the investigation of concepts of health and empowerment, with the goal of helping to inform and advance future theorizations and empirical enquiry in this field.

As previously described, my own interest in young people's health has been concerned with the marginalization of their perspectives and the broader tendency to problematize and pathologize young people and their health. This position may well explain why young people appeared to take up (and criticize) some discourses more readily than others (cf. Allen 2003a) or perhaps revealed a personal tendency to produce a more 'romanticized' view of young people. Likewise, my concern for issues of power and empowerment may have similarly contributed to my sensitivity to instances of contestation and resistance within the school context whilst unknowingly downplaying the potential significance of the more mundane, everyday encounters and interactions that take place between young people and adults.

A further note of caution is offered with respect to the groups of young people involved in the study. Arguably, evidence of the more positive and counter-hegemonic discourses of health found in this one study could be indicative of a form of sampling bias whereby the sample of young people represented a relatively motivated and health-conscious risk-averse group, or indeed, findings of this kind could be a consequence of the decision to focus on young people's accounts of 'feeling well'. On reflection, this focus on 'wellness' may have produced a set of responses that largely captured elements of young people's 'mental health' or their well-being, more so than a focus on physical aspects of health. This perhaps explains why young people appeared to place greater emphasis on those affective states of 'being happy', for example, rather than areas of physical health, such as obesity, smoking and drinking alcohol.

Despite these concerns, examining young people's accounts did highlight their sharp criticisms of the ways in which young people's health (in terms of smoking, drinking alcohol and unprotected sex) are currently presented and portrayed in health promotion policy and practice. Indeed, during fieldwork, young people sought repeatedly to distance themselves from these dominant discourses on health by emphasizing the more positive dimensions of their everyday lives (see Chapter Five). Although these findings may be understood as procedural limitations to interview guides, this study did elicit important discussions from young people about how these same negative discourses were thought to adversely affect their own health (see

Chapter Six). Indeed, young people themselves did discuss aspects of physical health, crucially drawing links between the physical and affective dimensions of health (see Chapter Five).

The more open-ended interview schedules thus enabled a more authentic account of young people's perspectives to be generated, which often revealed their criticisms of official health discourses. These criticisms might have been more difficult to identify and capture in a more heavily structured approach to data collection or by explicitly drawing on the term *health*. The decision to ask respondents about their thoughts in relation to 'feeling well' can be thus seen as one useful technique to help minimize any risk of priming responses around official perspectives on health.

Whilst this (more positive) approach to examining young people's health has revealed the varying ways health is differentially defined, understood and experienced (Blaxter 2010), a final note of caution is offered here. The multiple ways in which the concept of health has been conceptualized creates some difficulties for understanding health in terms of 'official' and 'alternative' perspectives as the conceptual framework for empowerment somewhat suggests. Arguably, both official and young people's alternative perspectives can be seen to capture a broad range of understandings of health, which may well reflect varying degrees, or a combination, of these broadly categorized perspectives. However, the newly developed framework on empowerment does offer potential to further scrutinize this conceptual 'muddiness' by drawing attention to (and further interrogating) how the conceptually distinct forms of empowerment may arise from (or give rise to) differing (and potentially competing) understandings of health.

By offering a new framework for understanding empowerment, an investigation of this kind has not only highlighted the importance of developing more responsive approaches to the promotion of young people's health but further opens up some new future directions (and challenges) for conceptual development, empirical enquiry and health promotion practice in support of young people's health.

Notes

Foreword

1 I am grateful to Claire Greslé-Favier for alerting me to the importance of this work.

Preface

1 See *Choosing Health: Making Healthy Choices Easier* (DH 2004a, chapter 3) for an example of protectionist and participatory discourses on young people's health. This chapter sets out the former UK Labour Government's action to protect young people's health through developing young people's knowledge and skills to responsibly manage their 'risky' health-related behaviours.

1 Introduction

1 *Ice* is a common street name for the drug crystal methamphetamine.
2 In the United Kingdom, the Labour Government was in office from May 1997 to May 2010.
3 On May 11, 2010, in the United Kingdom, a new Conservative–Liberal Democrat coalition government came into office.

2 The diverse meanings of empowerment

1 *Social capital* has many meanings and interpretations but is often referred to as being the (economic, political, social) resources available to an individual to act in line with his or her interests as a consequence of his or her positioning within the social structure (see Putnam 1995 and Bourdieu 1990, 1993).

3 Power, empowerment and young people

1 *Power to* interpretations draw on Machiavellian (1958 [original 1517]) notions of power and more recent 'agency' perspectives (see for example Archer 1988, McNay 2000, 2003).
2 *Power within* interpretations draw on components of psychological and self-empowerment, including the development of self-esteem and personal control (see Rissel 1994, Labonte 1996, Rowlands 1998) and existentialist approaches and the spirituality literature (see Craib 1976, Moss 2005).
3 *Power over* interpretations characterize structuralist perspectives including functionalist (see for example Parsons, 1967), Marxist (see for example Miliband 1969, Poulantzas 1976) and Marxist and radical feminist (see for example Harstock 1983, Young 1990).

4 *Power through* interpretations are indicated in ideological (see Gramsci 1971) and poststructuralist perspectives, most notably drawing on the work of Foucault (1980, 1990).

5 Pluralist perspectives point to the diversity of competing interest groups that hold varying degrees of power. Classical pluralist thought viewed power as dispersed between different social groups and becomes evident within decision-making processes as agency is exercised. Power is therefore seen as fixed within a zero-sum capacity so that if one group accumulates power it does so at the expense of another.

6 *Praxis* refers to reflection and action against oppression. Freire's (1970) interpretation of the concept is discussed later in the chapter.

7 The sociology of childhood examines the ways in which societies understand and organize childhood. This body of literature is underpinned by three key arguments. First, childhood is socially, rather biologically, constructed and reflects the attitudes, beliefs and values of a particular society at a particular time. Second, children and young people are considered to be social actors, contributing to the construction of social reality. Third, the social order is defined by a 'generational order' whereby members of society are categorized and organized on the basis of age (see James and Prout 1997, Mayall 2002, Jenks 2005, Qvortrup, Cosaro and Honig 2009).

8 Giddens's (1987, 1991) structuration theory also examines the relationship between structure and agency. According to Giddens, social structures are situated within human actions, which in turn produce and reproduce social structure and action. Consequently, human action is as inextricably linked to power as power is to agency.

9 Habermas's (1970) theory of communicative action is the means through which critical reflection and consciousness can be raised through the process of dialogue. This therapeutic dialogue develops resistance to the internalized distorted communication (ideology) that oppressed and marginalized groups experience and thus initiate and affect a process of emancipation and social change. Such forms of therapeutic dialogue therefore point to possibilities for consciousness-raising, similar to that of Freire's notion of *conscientização*, and the potential for empowerment to effect wider social structures.

10 Lukes's 1974 edition of *Power: A Radical View* examined existing debates on power at that time, including Dahl's (1957) agency model and theories linked to forms of decision-making (first dimension) and (based on Bachrach and Baratz's [1962] critique of Dahl) examining 'what does not happen' or the processes of agenda-setting (second dimension) Swartz 2007). However, his principal contribution was that of the third dimension and the conceptualization of ideological forms of power, which shaped subsequent thinking on power. Lukes thus ranked these dimensions in order of importance, the third being most fundamental as ideological forms of power come to shape the first and second dimensions. His later work, published in 2005, attended to criticisms of his 1974 book. Whilst remaining concerned with domination, in his most recent edition, Lukes integrated more recent contributions from Foucault and Bourdieu to highlight some of the more productive, dynamic and transformative potentials of power.

4 The study

1 An 'emic' research approach provides an account of the everyday meanings given to behaviours, beliefs and actions as described by participants themselves. In contrast, an 'etic' research approach derives more strongly from the terms of reference described by the researcher (Creswell 2012).

2 The sixth form centre offers postcompulsory education for young people between the ages of 16 and 18 years.
3 GCSE is the General Certificate of Secondary Education awarded in secondary schools in England, Wales and Northern Ireland.
4 Ofsted is the Office for Standards in Education, Children's Services and Schools (Ofsted) in England. Ofsted regulates and inspects the quality of educational provision in England, including those in all state-run schools.
5 The National Healthy Schools Programme (NHSP) was introduced in 1999 by the then Department of Children, Schools and Families and Department of Health in England. The main aim of the NHSP is to improve health, raise pupil achievement, improve social inclusion and encourage closer working between health and education sectors. The Healthy School Status is awarded to schools meeting and achieving a number of criteria.
6 See Gådin and Hammarström (2000) and Allen (2003a and b) for some exceptions.
7 Researchers engaging in forms of covert research often attempt to gain membership into the group under investigation (see Humphreys 1975, Ditton 1977).

5 Being happy and having fun

1 A previous version of this chapter (see Spencer 2013b) has been published in the journal *Health Education*. This chapter has been republished with full permission from the Emerald Publishing Group Limited.
2 To maintain anonymity, all names and identifying contextual features have been changed throughout.
3 A *hoodie* is a sweatshirt with a hood. In the 2000s, the hoodie has been associated with criminal and antisocial behaviour.
4 A *flat peak* is a hat where the peak has to be completely flat (Americans call these baseball caps or trucker hats).
5 *Chav* is a pejorative epithet referring to an individual usually associated with a working-class youth subculture in Britain.

7 Young people's priorities for health promotion

1 The school council and school parliament are committee groups set up by the school to enable young people to express their opinions and influence decisions at school (see Alderson 2000).

8 Empowerment and its relationship to young people's health

1 An earlier version of this chapter has been previously published in *Health: An Interdisciplinary Journal for the Social Study of Health, Illness and Medicine* (Spencer 2013a). This revised version is being republished with full permission from SAGE Publications Limited.

References

Abbott, D. A. and Dalla, R. L. (2008). 'It's a choice, simple as that: youth reasoning for sexual abstinence or activity'. *Journal of Youth Studies*, 11 (6), 629–649.

Abbott-Chapman, J., Denholm, C. and Wyld, C. (2008). 'Gender differences in adolescent risk-taking: are they diminishing?: An Australian Intergenerational Study'. *Youth and Society*, 40 (1), 131–154.

Abel, T. (2008). 'Cultural capital and social inequality in health'. *Journal of Epidemiology and Community Health*, 62 (7), 1–5.

Abel, T. and Frohlich, K. L. (2012). 'Capitals and capabilities: Linking structure and agency to reduce health inequalities'. *Social Science and Medicine*, 74 (2), 236–244.

Abercrombie, N., Hill, S. and Turner, B. S. (1980). *The Dominant Ideology Thesis*. London, UK: Allen and Unwin.

Acheson, D. (1998). *Independent Inquiry into Inequalities in Health: A Report*. London, UK: TSO.

Agar, M. H. (1996). 'Recasting the "ethno" in "epidemiology"'. *Medical Anthropology*, 16 (4), 391–403.

Aggleton, P. (1987). *Rebels Without a Cause? Middle Class Youth and the Transition from School to Work*. London, UK: Falmer Press.

Aggleton, P. and Campbell, C. (2000). 'Working with young people – towards an agenda for sexual health'. *Sexual and Relationship Therapy*, 15 (3), 283–296.

Aggleton, P., Rivers, K., Mulvihill, C., Chase, E., Downie, A., Sinkler, P., Tyrer, P. and Warwick, I. (2000). 'Lessons learned: working towards the National Healthy School Standard'. *Health Education*, 100 (3), 102–110.

Aggleton, P. and Whitty, G. (1985). 'Rebels without a cause? Socialization and subcultural style among the children of the new middle classes'. *Sociology of Education*, 58 (1), 60–72.

Aggleton, P., Whitty, G., Knight, A., Prayle, D. and Warwick, I. (1996). *Promoting Young People's Health: The Health Concerns and Needs of Young People*. London, UK: Health Education Research Unit, Institute of Education.

Aggleton, P., Whitty, G., Knight, A., Prayle, D., Warwick, I. and Rivers, K. (1998). 'Promoting young people's health: the health concerns and needs of young people'. *Health Education*, 98 (6), 213–219.

Aguinaldo, J. P. (2004). 'Rethinking validity in qualitative research from a social constructionist perspective: from "is this valid research?" to "what is this research valid for?"'. *Qualitative Report*, 9 (1), 127–136.

Ajzen, I. and Fishbein, M. (1980). *Understanding Attitudes and Predicting Social Behaviour*. Englewood Cliffs, NJ: Prentice-Hall.

Alanen, L. (2001). 'Explorations in generational analysis'. In L. Alanen and B. Mayall (eds.). *Conceptualizing Child–Adult Relations*. London, UK: Routledge Falmer. pp. 11–23.

Alanen, L. and Mayall, B. (eds.) (2001). *Conceptualizing Child–Adult Relations*. London, UK: Routledge Falmer.

Alderson, P. (2000). 'School students' views on school councils and daily life at school'. *Children and Society*, 14 (2), 121–134.

Alderson, P. (2008). 'Children as researchers: participation rights and research methods'. In P. Christensen and A. James (eds.). *Research with Children: Perspectives and Practices*. New York, NY: Routledge Falmer. pp. 276–291.

Alderson, P. and Morrow, V. (2011). *Ethics, Social Research and Consulting with Children and Young People*. (2nd ed). London, UK: Sage.

Alexander, S. A. C., Frochlich, K. L., Poland, B. D., Haines, R. J. and Maule, C. (2010). ' "I'm a young student, I'm a girl . . . and for some reason they are hard on me for smoking": the role of gender and social context for smoking behaviour'. *Critical Public Health*, 20 (3), 323–338.

Alinsky, S. (1989). *Reveille for Radicals*. New York, NY: Vintage Books.

Allen, L. (2003a). 'Girls want sex, boys want love: resisting dominant discourses of (hetero)sexuality'. *Sexualities*, 6 (2), 215–236.

———. (2003b). 'Power talk: young people negotiating (hetero)sex'. *Women's Studies International Forum*, 26 (3), 235–244.

———. (2007). 'Denying the sexual subject: schools' regulation of student sexuality'. *British Educational Research Journal*, 33 (2), 221–234.

———. (2008). 'Young people's "agency" in sexuality research using visual methods'. *Journal of Youth Studies*, 11 (6), 565–577.

Altheide, D. L. and Johnson, J. M. (2013). 'Reflections on interpretive adequacy in qualitative research'. In N. K. Denzin and Y. S. Lincoln (eds.). *Collecting and Interpreting Qualitative Materials*. Thousand Oaks, CA: Sage. pp. 381–413.

Althusser, L. (1971). *Lenin and Philosophy and Other Essays*. London, UK: New Left Books.

Altman, D. G. and Feighery, E. C. (2004). 'Future directions for youth empowerment: commentary on application of youth empowerment theory to tobacco control'. *Health Education and Behaviour*, 31 (5), 641–647.

Amos, A. and Bostock, Y. (2007). 'Young people, smoking and gender – a qualitative exploration'. *Health Education Research*, 22 (6), 770–781.

Anderson, J. M. (1996). 'Empowering patients: issues and strategies'. *Social Science and Medicine*, 43 (5), 697–705.

Angrosino, M. (2007). *Doing Ethnographic and Observational Research*. London, UK: Sage.

Antonovsky, A. (1979). *Health, Stress and Coping*. San Francisco, CA: Jossey-Bass.

Arai, L. (2009). *Teenage Pregnancy: The Making and Unmaking of a Problem*. Bristol, UK: Policy Press.

Archer, L., Hollingworth, S. and Halsall, A. (2007). ' "University's not for me – I'm a Nike person": urban, working-class young people's negotiations of "style", identity and educational engagement'. *Sociology*, 41 (2), 219–237.

Archer, M. S. (1988). *Culture and Agency. The Place of Culture in Social Theory*. Cambridge, UK: Cambridge University Press.

Armstrong, C., Hill, M. and Secker, J. (2000). 'Young people's perceptions of mental health'. *Children and Society,* 14 (1), 60–72.

Armstrong, N. and Murphy, E. (2011). 'Conceptualizing resistance'. *Health,* 16 (3), 314–326.

Ashcraft, C. (2006). 'Ready or not . . .? Teen sexuality and the troubling discourse of readiness'. *Anthropology and Education Quarterly,* 37 (4), 328–346.

Ashton, J. and Seymour, H. (1988). *The New Public Health.* Buckingham, UK: Open University Press.

Ashworth, P. D., Longmate, M. A. and Morrison, P. (1992). 'Patient participation: its meaning and significance in the context of caring'. *Journal of Advanced Nursing,* 17 (12), 1430–1439.

Ataöv, A. and Haider, J. (2006). 'From participation to empowerment: critical reflections on a participatory action research project with street children in Turkey'. *Children, Youth and Environments,* 16 (2), 127–152.

Austen, L. (2009). 'The social construction of risk by young people'. *Health, Risk and Society,* 11 (5), 451–470.

Australian Government. (2010). *National Strategy for Young Australians.* [Online]. Available at http://www.youth.gov.au/sites/Youth/bodyImage/Documents/NatStrat .pdf [Last accessed 23rd April 2013].

Australian Institute of Health and Welfare [AIHW]. (2011). *Young Australians: Their Health and Well-Being 2011.* [Online]. Available at: http://www.aihw.gov .au/WorkArea/DownloadAsset.aspx?id=10737419259 [Last accessed 23rd April 2013].

Aynsley-Green, A., Barker, M., Burr, S., MacFarlane, A., Morgan, J., Sibert, J., Turner, T., Viner, R., Waterson, T. and Hall, D. (2000). 'Who is speaking for children and adolescents and for their health at the policy level?' *British Medical Journal,* 321 (7255), 229–232.

Bachrach, P. and Baratz, M. S. (1962). 'Two faces of power'. *American Political Science Review,* 56 (4), 947–952.

Bagnoli, A. and Clark, A. (2010). 'Focus groups with young people: a participatory approach to research planning'. *Journal of Youth Studies,* 13 (1), 101–119.

Baillie, L., Lovato, C. Y., Johnson, J. L. and Kalaw, C. (2005). 'Smoking decisions from a teen perspective: a narrative study'. *American Journal of Health Behaviour,* 29 (2), 99–106.

Baker, J. (2008). 'The ideology of choice. Overstating progress and hiding injustice in the lives of young women: findings from a study in North Queensland, Australia'. *Women's Studies International Forum,* 31 (1), 53–64.

Balen, R., Blyth, E., Calabretto, H., Fraser, C., Horrocks, C. and Manby, M. (2006). 'Involving children in health and social research: "human becomings" or "active beings"?' *Childhood,* 13 (1), 29–48.

Bandura, A. (1977). 'Self-efficacy theory: toward a unifying theory of behaviour change'. *Psychological Review,* 84 (2), 191–215.

———. (1982). 'Self-efficacy mechanisms in human agency'. *American Psychologist,* 37 (2), 122–147.

Barber, T. (2007). 'Young people and civic participation: a conceptual review'. *Youth and Policy,* 96: 19–39.

Barker, C. (1999). 'Empowerment and resistance: "collective effervescence" and other accounts'. In P. Bagguley and J. Hearn (eds.). *Transforming Politics: Power and Resistance.* Basingstoke, UK: Macmillan Press. pp. 11–31.

Barker, J. and Weller, S. (2003). 'Never work with children?: the geography of methodological issues in research with children'. *Qualitative Research*, 3 (2), 207–227.

Barnes, C. and Mercer, G. (1995). 'Disability: emancipation, community participation and disabled people'. In G. Craig and M. Mayo (eds.). *Community Empowerment: A Reader in Participation and Development*. London, UK: Zed Books. pp. 33–45.

Bartky, S. (1990). *Femininity and Domination: Studies in the Phenomenology of Oppression*. New York, NY: Routledge.

Bauer, K. W., Yang, W. Y. and Austin, B. S. (2004). ' "How can we stay healthy when you're throwing all of this in front of us?" Findings from focus groups and interviews in middle schools on environmental influences on nutrition and physical activity'. *Health Education and Behaviour*, 31 (1), 34–46.

Bauman, Z. (1996). 'From pilgrim to tourist – a short history of identity'. In S. Hall and P. duGay (eds.). *Questions of Cultural Identity*. London, UK: Sage. pp. 18–37.

Baxter, J. (2002). 'Competing discourses in the classroom: a Post-Structuralist discourse analysis of girls' and boys' speech in public contexts'. *Discourse and Society*, 13 (6), 827–842.

Bennett, E. and Gough, B. (2013). 'In pursuit of leanness: the management of appearance, affect and masculinities within a men's weight loss forum'. *Health*, 17 (3), 284–299.

Berg, M., Coman, E. and Schensul, J. J. (2009). 'Youth action research for prevention: a multi-level intervention designed to increase efficacy and empowerment among urban youth'. *American Journal of Community Psychology*, 43 (3–4), 345–359.

Berman, H. (2003). 'Getting critical with children: empowering approaches with a disempowered group'. *Advances in Nursing Science*, 10 (49), 102–113.

Bernstein, B. (1977). *Class, Codes and Control*. (Vol. 3). London, UK: Routledge and Kegan Paul.

———. (1982). 'Class, modalities and the process of cultural reproduction: a model'. In M. Apple (ed.). *Codes, Modalities and the Process of Cultural Reproduction*. London, UK: Routledge and Kegan Paul. pp. 304–355.

———. (1990). *Class, Codes and Control: The Structuring of Pedagogic Discourse*. (vol. 4). London, UK: Routledge and Kegan Paul.

Bernstein, E., Wallerstein, N., Braithwaite, R., Gutierrez, L., Labonte, R. and Zimmerman, M. (1994). 'Empowerment forum: a dialogue between guest editorial board members'. *Health Education Quarterly*, 21 (3), 281–294.

Bishai, D. M., Mercer, D. and Tapales, A. (2005). 'Can government policies help adolescents avoid risky behaviour?' *Preventive Medicine*, 40 (2), 197–202.

Bjerke, H. (2011). ' "It's the way they do it": Expressions of agency in child-adult relations at home and school'. *Children and Society*, 25 (2), 93–103.

Blackman, S. J. (2007). 'Hidden ethnography: crossing emotional borders in qualitative accounts of young people's lives'. *Sociology*, 41 (4), 699–716.

Blaikie, N. (2007). *Approaches to Social Enquiry*. (2nd ed.). Cambridge, UK: Polity Press.

Blanchard, A. K., Mohan, H. L., Shahmanesh, M., Prakash, R., Isac, S., Ramesh, B. M., Bhattacharjee, P., Gurnani, V., Moses, S. and Blanchard J. F. (2013). 'Community mobilization, empowerment and HIV prevention among female sex workers in south India'. *BMC Public Health*, 16 (13), 234–247.

Blaxter, M. (2010). *Health*. (2nd ed.). Cambridge, UK: Polity Press.

Bloor, M., Frankland, J., Thomas, M. and Robson, K. (2004). *Focus Groups in Social Research*. London, UK: Sage.

Bogren, A. (2006). 'The competent drinker, the authentic person and the strong person: reasoning in Swedish young people's discussions about alcohol'. *Journal of Youth Studies*, 9 (5), 515–538.

Bordo, S. (1993). *Unbearable Weight: Feminism, Western Culture and the Body*. Los Angeles: University of California Press.

Bourdieu, P. (1990). *The Logic of Practice*. Cambridge, UK: Polity Press.

———. (1991). *Language and Symbolic Power*. Cambridge, UK: Polity Press.

———. (1993). *The Field of Cultural Production*. Cambridge, UK: Polity Press.

Boylan, J. and Ing, P. (2005). 'Seen but not heard—young people's experience of advocacy'. *International Journal of Social Welfare*, 14 (1), 2–12.

Bradbury-Jones, C. Sambrook, S. and Irvine, F. (2008). 'Power and empowerment in nursing: a fourth theoretical approach'. *Journal of Advanced Nursing*, 62 (2), 258–266.

Braunack-Mayer, A. and Louise, J. (2008). 'The ethics of community empowerment: Tensions in health promotion theory and practice'. *Promotion and Education*, 15 (3), 5–8.

Brewer, J.D. (2005). *Ethnography: Understanding Social Research*. Buckingham, UK: Open University Press.

Briggs, D. (2010). 'True stories from bare times on the road: developing empowerment, identity and social capital among urban minority ethnic young people in London, UK'. *Ethnic and Racial Studies*, 33 (5), 851–871.

Brooks, F. and Magnusson, J. (2007). 'Physical activity as leisure: the meaning of physical activity for the health and well-being of adolescent women'. *Health Care for Women International*, 28 (1), 69–87.

Bryman, A. (2012). *Social Research Methods*. (4th ed.). Oxford, UK: Oxford University Press.

Busseri, M.A., Willoughby, T. and Chalmers, H. (2007). 'A rationale and method for examining reasons for linkages among adolescent risk behaviours'. *Journal of Youth and Adolescence*, 36 (3), 279–289.

Butler, U.M. and Princeswal, M. (2010). 'Cultures of participation: young people's engagement in the public sphere in Brazil'. *Community Development Journal*, 45 (3), 335–345.

Cameron, E., Mathers, J. and Parry, J. (2008). 'Health and well-being: questioning the use of health concepts in public health policy and practice'. *Critical Public Health*, 18 (2), 225–232.

Campbell, C. (2009). 'Distinguishing the power of agency from agentic power: a note on Weber and the "Black Box" of personal agency'. *Sociological Theory*, 27 (4), 407–418.

Campbell, C. and MacPhail, C. (2002). 'Peer education, gender and the development of critical consciousness: participatory HIV prevention by South African youth'. *Social Science and Medicine*, 55 (2), 331–345.

Campos, P., Saguy, A., Ernsberger, P., Oliver, E. and Gaesser, G. (2006). 'The epidemiology of overweight and obesity: public health crisis or moral panic?' *International Journal of Epidemiology*, 35 (1), 55–60.

Cavet, J. and Sloper, P. (2004). 'The participation of children and young people in decisions about UK service development'. *Child: Care, Health and Development*, 30 (6), 613–621.

Chabot, C., Shoveller, J. E., Spencer, G. and Johnson, J. L. (2012). 'Ethical and epistemological insights: a case study of participatory action research with young people'. *Journal of Empirical Research on Human Research Ethics*, 7 (2), 20–33.

Chang, L., Li, I. and Liu, C. (2004). 'A study of the empowerment process for cancer patients using Freire's dialogical interviewing'. *Journal of Nursing Research*, 12 (1), 41–50.

Chang, L., Liu, C. and Yen, E. (2008). 'Effects of an empowerment-based education program for public health nurses in Taiwan'. *Journal of Clinical Nursing*, 17 (20), 2782–2790.

Charles, N. and Walters, V. (2008). 'Men are leavers alone and women are worriers: gender differences in discourses of health'. *Health, Risk and Society*, 10 (2), 117–132.

Chawla, L., Blanchet-Cohen, N., Cosco, N., Driskell, D., Krueger, J., Malone, K., Moore, P. and Percy-Smith, B. (2005). ' "Don't just listen – do something!" Lessons learnt about governance from the Growing up in Cities project'. *Children, Youth and Environments*, 15 (2), 53–88.

Christensen, P. and James, A. (eds.) (2008). *Research with Children: Perspectives and Practices*. (2nd ed.). Abingdon, UK: Routledge.

Christensen, P. and Prout, A. (2002). 'Working with ethical symmetry in social research with children'. *Childhood*, 9 (4), 477–497.

Clarke, J., Hall, S., Jefferson, T. and Roberts, B. (1976). 'Subcultures, cultures and class'. In S. Hall and T. Jefferson (eds.). *Resistance through Rituals: Youth Subcultures in Post-War Britain*. Abingdon, UK: Routledge. pp. 3–59.

Clatts, M. C. and Sotheran, J. L. (2000). 'Challenges in research on drug and sexual risk practices of men who have sex with men: applications of ethnography in HIV epidemiology and prevention'. *AIDS and Behaviour*, 4 (2), 169–179.

Clegg, S. R. (1998). *Frameworks of Power*. London, UK: Sage.

Clegg, S. (2006). 'The problem of agency in feminism: a critical realist approach'. *Gender and Education*, 18 (3), 309–324.

Coe, A-B., Goicolea, I., Hurtig, A-K. and Sebastian, M. S. (2012). 'Understanding how young people do activism: youth strategies on sexual health in Ecuador and Peru'. *Youth and Society*. Advance online publication. doi:10.1177/0044118X12464640.

Colic-Peisker, V. (2004). 'Doing ethnography in "one's own ethnic community": the experience of an awkward insider'. In L. Hume and J. Mulcock (eds.). *Anthropologists in the Field: Cases in Participant Observation*. New York, NY: Columbia University Press. pp. 82–95.

Connell, R. W. (2005). *Masculinities*. (2nd ed.). Cambridge, UK: Polity Press.

Cook, D. T. (2007). 'The disempowering empowerment of children's consumer "choice": cultural discourses of the child consumer in North America'. *Society and Business Review*, 2 (1), 37–52.

Courtney, W. H. (2000). 'Constructions of masculinity and their influence on men's well-being: a theory of gender and health'. *Social Science and Medicine*, 50 (10), 1385–1401.

Craib, I. (1976). *Existentialism and Sociology*. Cambridge, UK: Cambridge University Press.

Crawford, R. (2004). 'Risk ritual and the management of control and anxiety in medical culture'. *Health*, 8 (4), 505–528.

Cree, V.E., Helen, K. and Tisdall, K. (2002). 'Research with children: sharing the dilemmas'. *Children and Family Social Work*, 7 (1), 47–56.

Creswell, J.W. (2012). *Qualitative Inquiry and Research Design: Choosing Among Five Traditions*. (3rd ed.). Thousand Oaks, CA: Sage.

Croll, J.K., Neumark-Sztainer, D. and Story, M. (2001). 'Healthy eating: what does it mean to adolescents?' *Journal of Nutrition Education*, 33 (4), 193–198.

Crossley, M.L. (2001a). 'The Armistead project: an exploration of gay men, sexual practices, community health promotion and issues of empowerment'. *Journal of Community and Applied Social Psychology*, 11 (2), 111–123.

———. (2001b). 'Resistance and health promotion'. *Health Education Journal*, 60 (3), 197–204.

———. (2002). '"Could you please pass one of those health leaflets along?" Exploring health, morality and resistance through focus groups'. *Social Science and Medicine*, 55 (8), 1471–1483.

Currie, D.H., Kelly, D.M. and Pomerantz, S. (2006). 'The geeks shall inherit the earth: girls' agency, subjectivity and empowerment'. *Journal of Youth Studies*, 9 (4), 419–436.

———. (2011). 'Skater girlhood: resignifying femininism'. In R. Gill and C. Scharff (eds.). *New Femininities: Postfeminism, Neoliberalism and Subjectivity*. Basingstoke, UK: Palgrave Macmillan. pp. 293–306.

Curtis, K., Liabo, K., Roberts, H. and Barker, M. (2004). 'Consulted but not heard: a qualitative study of young people's views of their local health service'. *Health Expectations*, 7 (2), 149–156.

Curtis, S. (1992). 'Promoting health through a developmental analysis of adolescent risk behaviour'. *Journal of School Health*, 62 (9), 417–420.

Curtis, S. and Jones, I. R. (1998). 'Is there a place for geography in the analysis of health inequality?' *Sociology of Health and Illness*, 20 (5), 645-672.

Dahl, R.A. (1957). 'The concept of power'. *Behavioural Science*, 2 (3), 201–215.

Dahlgren, G. and Whitehead, M. (1991). 'Tackling inequalities: a review of policy initiatives'. In M. Benzeval, K. Judge and M. Whitehead (eds.). *Tackling Inequalities in Health: An Agenda for Action*. London, UK: Kings Fund Institute. pp. 22–52.

Dalrymple, J. (2001). 'Safeguarding young people through confidential advocacy services'. *Child and Family Social Work*, 6 (2), 149–162.

Darbyshire, P., MacDougall, C. and Schiller, W. (2005). 'Multiple methods in qualitative research with children: more insight or just more?' *Qualitative Research*, 5 (4), 417–436.

Data Protection Act. (1998). London, UK: HMSO. [Online]. Available at: http://www.legislation.gov.uk/ukpga/1998/29/contents [Last accessed 18th April 2013].

David, M., Edwards, R. and Alldred, P. (2001). 'Children and school-based research: "informed consent" or "educated consent"?' *British Educational Research Journal*, 27 (3), 347–365.

Delp, L., Brown, M. and Domenzain, A. (2005). 'Fostering youth leadership to address workplace and community environmental health issues: a university-school-community partnership'. *Health Promotion Practice*, 6 (3), 270–285.

Denscombe, M. (2000). 'Peer group pressure, young people and smoking: new developments and policy implications'. *Drugs: Education, Prevention and Policy*, 8 (1), 1–26.

———. (2001a). 'Critical incidents and the perception of health risks: the experiences of young people in relation to their use of alcohol and tobacco'. *Health, Risk and Society*, 3 (3), 293–306.

———. (2001b). 'Uncertain identities and health-risking behaviour: the case of young people and smoking in late modernity'. *British Journal of Sociology, 52* (1), 157–177.

Dentith, A.M., Measor, L. and O'Malley, M.P. (2009). 'Stirring dangerous waters: dilemmas for critical participatory research with young people'. *Sociology, 43* (1), 158–168.

Denzin, N. (2007). *On Understanding Emotion.* (2nd ed.). New Brunswick, NJ: Transaction.

Denzin, N. and Lincoln, Y.S. (eds.). (2011). *The SAGE Handbook of Qualitative Research.* Thousand Oaks, CA: Sage.

Department for Children, Schools and Families [DCSF]. (2007). *Aiming High for Young People: A Ten Year Strategy for Positive Activities.* London, UK: DCSF.

Department for Education [DfE]. (2013). *School and Local Statistics.* [Online]. Available at: http://www.education.gov.uk/cgi-bin/schools/performance/school [Last accessed 23rd April 2013].

Department for Education and Skills [DfES]. (2003). *Every Child Matters.* London, UK: DfES.

Department for Education and Skills/Department of Health [DfES/DH]. (2005). *National Healthy School Status: A Guide for Schools.* London, UK: DfES/DH.

———. (2006). *Youth Matters: Next Steps.* London, UK: DfES.

Department of Health [DH]. (1992). *The Health of the Nation: A Strategy for Health for England.* London, UK: TSO.

———. (1999). *Saving Lives: Our Healthier Nation.* London, UK: TSO.

———. (2004a). *Choosing Health: Making Healthy Choices Easier.* London, UK: TSO.

———. (2004b). *National Service Framework for Children, Young People and Maternity Services.* London, UK: TSO.

———. (2006). *Our Health, Our Care, Our Say: A New Direction for Community Services.* London, UK: TSO.

———. (2010a). *Equity and Excellence: Liberating the NHS.* London, UK: TSO.

———. (2010b). *Healthy Lives, Healthy People: Our Strategy for Public Health in England.* London, UK: TSO.

Department of Health/Department for Children, Schools and Families [DH/DCSF]. (2009). *Healthy Lives, Brighter Futures: The Strategy for Children and Young People's Health.* London, UK: TSO.

Devine, F. (2004). *Class Practices: How Parents Help Their Children Get Good Jobs.* Cambridge, UK: Cambridge University Press.

Devine, F., Savage, M., Scott, J. and Crompton, R. (eds.) (2005). *Rethinking Class: Culture, Identities and Lifestyle.* Basingstoke, UK: Palgrave Macmillan.

deVisser, R.O. and McDonnell, E.J. (2013). 'Man points: masculine capital and young men's health'. *Health Psychology, 32* (1), 5–14.

deWinter, M., Baerveldt, C. and Kooistra, J. (1999). 'Enabling children: participation as a new perspective on child-health promotion'. *Child, Health and Development, 25* (1), 15–25.

Dhand, A. (2007). 'Using learning theory to understand access in ethnographic research'. In G. Walford (ed.), *Studies in Educational Ethnography: Methodological Developments in Ethnography.* Bingley, UK: Emerald. pp. 1–27.

Ditton, J. (1977). *Part-time Crime: An Ethnography of Fiddling and Pilferage.* London, UK: Macmillan.

Dixey, R., Sahota, P., Atwal, S. and Turner, A. (2001). ' "Ha ha, you're fat, we're strong": a qualitative study of boys' and girls' perceptions of fatness, thinness, social pressures and health using focus groups'. *Health Education*, 101 (5), 206–216.

Doull, M. (2009). *Girl Power/Boy Power: Positive Sexual Health Outcomes and Gendered Dynamics of Power in Adolescent Heterosexual Relationships*. Unpublished doctoral dissertation. University of Ottawa, Ottawa, Ontario, Canada.

Doull, M. and Sethna, C. (2011). 'Subject, object or both? Defining the boundaries of girl power'. *Girlhood Studies*, 4 (2), 92–110.

Duff, C. (2003). 'The importance of culture and context: rethinking risk and risk management in young drug using populations'. *Health, Risk and Society*, 5 (3), 285–299.

Duits, L. and van Zoonen, L. (2006). 'Headscarves and porno-chic: disciplining girls' bodies in the European multicultural society'. *European Journal of Women's Studies*, 13 (2), 103–117.

Duncan, P. (2004). 'Dispute, dissent and the place of health promotion in a "disrupted tradition" of health improvement'. *Public Understanding of Science*, 13 (2), 177–190.

Duncan, P. (2007). *Critical Perspectives on Health*. Basingstoke, UK: Palgrave Macmillan.

Duncan, P. and Cribb, A. (1996). 'Helping people change – an ethical approach?' *Health Education Research*, 11 (3), 339–348.

Duncan, R. E., Drew, S. E., Hodgson, J. and Sawyer, S. M. (2009). ' "Is my mum going to hear this"? Methodological and ethical challenges in qualitative health research with young people'. *Social Science and Medicine*, 69, (11), 1691–1699.

Duncombe, J. and Jessop, J. (2012). ' "Doing rapport" and the ethics of "faking friendship" '. In M. Mauthner, M. Birch, J. Jessop and T. Miller (eds.). *Ethics in Qualitative Research*. (2nd ed.). London, UK: Sage. pp. 108–122.

Dworkski-Riggs, D. and Langhout, R. D. (2010). 'Elucidating the power in empowerment and the participation in Participatory Action Research: a story about a research team and elementary school change'. *American Journal of Community Psychology*, 45 (3–4), 215–230.

Emler, N. (2001). *Self-Esteem: The Costs and Causes of Low Self-Worth*. York, UK: Joseph Rowntree Foundation.

Essau, C. A. (2004). 'Risk-taking behaviour among German adolescents'. *Journal of Youth Studies*, 7 (4), 499–512.

European Network for Health Promoting Schools [ENHPS]. (2005). *The Health Promoting School: International Advances in Theory, Evaluation and Practice*. Copenhagen, Denmark: WHO Regional Office for Europe. [Online]. Available at: http://www.euro.who.int/__data/assets/pdf_file/0012/111117/E90358.pdf [Last accessed 18th April 2013].

Evans, A., Riley, S. and Shankar, A. (2010). 'Technologies of sexiness: theorizing women's engagement in the sexualisation of culture'. *Feminism and Psychology*, 20 (1), 114–131.

Evans, J. and Davies, B. (2010). 'Family, class and embodiment: why school physical education makes so little difference to post-school participation patterns in physical activity'. *International Journal of Qualitative Studies in Education*, 23 (7), 765–784.

Eyben, R. and Napier-Moore, R. (2009). 'Choosing words with care? Shifting meanings of women's empowerment in international development'. *Third World Quarterly,* 30 (2), 285–300.

Ezzy, D. (2002). *Qualitative Analysis: Practice and Innovation.* London, UK: Routledge.

Farrant, W. (1991). 'Addressing the contradictions: health promotion and community health action in the United Kingdom'. *International Journal of Health Services,* 21 (3), 423–439.

Fields, E. L., Bogart, L. M., Smith, K. C., Malebranche, D. J., Ellen, J. and Schuster, M. A. (2012). 'HIV risk perceptions of masculinity among young black men who have sex with men'. *Journal of Adolescent Health,* 50 (3), 296–303.

Fletcher, K. (2006). 'Beyond dualism: leading out of oppression'. *Nursing Forum,* 41 (2), 50–59.

Flewitt, R. (2005). 'Conducting research with young children: some ethical considerations'. *Early Child Development and Care,* 175 (6), 553–565.

Foucault, M. (1980). *Power/Knowledge: Selected Interviews and Other Writings 1972–1977 by Michel Foucault.* [Trans. C. Gordon, L. Marshall, J. Mepham and K. Soper]. London, UK: Harvester Press.

———. (1988). 'Technologies of the self'. In L. Martin, H. Gutman and P. Hutton (eds.), *Technologies of the Self: A Seminar with Michael Foucault.* London, UK: Tavistock, 16–50.

———. (1990). *The Will to Knowledge: The History of Sexuality: Volume 1.* [Trans. R. Hurley]. London, UK: Penguin.

———. (1991). 'Governmentality'. In G. Burchell, C. Gordon and P. Miller (eds.). *The Foucault Effect: Studies in Governmentality.* Hemel Hempstead, UK: Harvester Wheatsheaf. pp. 87–105.

France, A. (2000). 'Towards a sociological understanding of youth and their risk-taking'. *Journal of Youth Studies,* 3 (3), 317–331.

———. (2004). 'Young people'. In S. Fraser, V. Lewis, S. Ding, M. Kellett and C. Robinson (eds.). *Doing Research with Children and Young People.* London, UK: Sage. pp. 175–191.

France, A., Bendelow, G. and Williams, S. (2000). 'A 'risky' business: researching the health beliefs of children and young people'. In A. Lewis and G. Lindsay (eds.). *Researching Children's Perspectives.* Buckingham, UK: Open University Press. pp. 150–163.

Fraser, S., Lewis, V., Ding, S., Kellett, M. and Robinson, C. (eds.) (2004). *Doing Research with Children and Young People.* London, UK: Sage.

Freire, P. (1970). *Pedagogy of the Oppressed.* New York, NY: Continuum.

Freire, P. (1996). *Pedagogy of the Oppressed.* (2nd ed.). London, UK: Penguin Books.

Frohlich, K. L., Corin, E. and Potvin, L. (2001). 'A theoretical proposal for the relationship between context and disease'. *Sociology of Health and Illness,* 23 (6), 776–797.

Frohlich, K. L., Potvin, L., Chabot, P. and Corin, E. (2002). 'A theoretical and empirical analysis of context: neighbourhoods, smoking and youth'. *Social Science and Medicine,* 54 (9), 1401–1417.

Gådin, K. G. and Hammarström, A. (2000). ' "We won't let them keep us quiet . . .":
Gendered strategies in the negotiation of power – implications for pupils' health and school health promotion'. *Health Promotion International,* 15 (4), 303–311.

Gaiswinkler, W. and Roessler, M. (2009). 'Using the expertise of knowing and the expertise of not-knowing to support processes of empowerment in social work practice'. *Journal of Social Work Practice*, 23 (2), 215–227.

Gallagher, U. and Burden, J. (1994). 'Nursing as health promotion: a myth accepted?' In J. Wilson-Barnett and J. Macleod-Clark (eds.). *Research in Health Promotion and Nursing*. London, UK: Macmillan. pp. 51–58.

Gavey, N. (2012). 'Beyond "empowerment"? Sexuality in a sexist world. *Sex Roles*, 66 (11–12), 718–724.

Gibson, C. (1991). 'A concept analysis of empowerment'. *Journal of Advanced Nursing*, 16 (3), 354–361.

Gibson, C. and Woolcock, M. (2008). 'Empowerment, deliberate development and local-level politics in Indonesia: participatory projects as a source of countervailing power'. *Studies in Comparative International Development*, 43 (2), 151–180.

Giddens, A. (1976a). 'Hermeneutics, ethnomethodology, and the problem of interpretive analysis'. In L. A. Coser and O. Larsen (eds.). *The Uses of Controversy in Sociology*. New York, NY: Basic Books. pp. 315–329.

———. (1976b). *New Rules of Sociological Method*. London, UK: Hutchinson.

———. (1987). *Social Theory and Modern Sociology*. Cambridge, UK: Polity Press.

———. (1991). *Modernity and Self Identity*. Cambridge, UK: Polity Press.

Gilbert, E. (2007). 'Constructing 'fashionable' youth identities: Australian young women cigarette smokers'. *Journal of Youth Studies*, 10 (1), 1–15.

Gilbert, T. (1995). 'Nursing: empowerment and the problem of power'. *Journal of Advanced Nursing*, 21 (5), 865–871.

Gill, A., Fitzgerald, S., Bhutani, S., Mand, H. and Sharma, S. (2010). 'The relationship between transformational leadership and employee desire for empowerment'. *International Journal of Contemporary Hospitality Management*, 22 (2), 263–273.

Gill, R. (2007a). 'Critical respect: The difficulties and dilemmas of agency and 'choice' for feminism: a reply to Duits and van Zoonen'. *European Journal of Women's Studies*, 14 (1), 69–80.

———. (2007b). 'Postfeminist media culture: elements of sensibility'. *European Journal of Cultural Studies*, 10 (2), 147–166.

———. (2008). 'Empowerment/sexism: figuring female sexual agency in contemporary advertising'. *Feminism and Psychology*, 18 (1), 35–60.

———. (2009). 'Beyond the "Sexualisation of Culture" thesis: an intersectional analysis of "sixpacks", "midriffs" and "hot lesbians" in advertising'. *Sexualities*, 12 (2), 137–160.

Gillham, B. (2008). *Observation Techniques: Structured to Unstructured*. London, UK: Continuum.

Gillman, M. (1996). 'Empowering professionals in higher education'. In B. Humphries (ed.). *Critical Perspectives on Empowerment*. Birmingham, UK: Venture Press. pp. 99–116.

Giroux, H. (1983). 'Theories of reproduction and resistance in the new sociology of education: a critical analysis'. *Harvard Educational Review*, 53 (3), 257–293.

Goldenberg, S., Shoveller, J., Koehoorn, M. and Ostry, A. (2008). 'Barriers to STI testing among youth in a Canadian oil and gas community'. *Health and Place*, 14 (4), 718–729.

Gomm, R. (1993). 'Issues of power in health and welfare'. In J. Walmsley, J. Reynolds, P. Shakespeare and R. Woolfe (eds.). *Health, Welfare and Practice*. London, UK: Sage. pp. 131–138.

Gordon, H. R. (2007). 'Allies within and without: how adolescent activists conceptualize ageism and navigate adult power in youth social movements'. *Journal of Contemporary Ethnography*, 36 (6), 631–668.

Gordon, J. and Turner, K. M. (2004). 'The empowerment principle: casualties of two schools' failure to grasp the nettle'. *Health Education*, 104 (4), 226–240.

Gosling, R., Stanistreet, D. and Swami, V. (2008). ' "If Michael Owen drinks it, why can't I?" 9 and 10 year olds perceptions of physical activity and healthy eating'. *Health Education Journal*, 67 (3), 167–181.

Grace, V. M. (1991). 'The marketing of empowerment and the construction of the health consumer: a critique of health promotion'. *International Journal of Health Services*, 21 (2), 329–343.

Gramsci, A. (1971). *Prison Notebooks*. (Vol. 1). New York, NY: Columbia University Press.

Grbich, C. (2012). *Qualitative Data Analysis: An Introduction*. (2nd ed.). London, UK: Sage.

Green, E., Mitchell, W. and Bunton, R. (2000). 'Contextualising risk and danger: an analysis of young people's perceptions of risk'. *Journal of Youth Studies*, 3 (2), 109–126.

Green, J. and Thorogood, N. (2009). *Qualitative Methods for Health Research*. (2nd ed.). London, UK: Sage.

Green, J. and Tones, K. (2010). *Health Promotion: Planning and Strategies*. (3rd ed.). London, UK: Sage.

Greene, S. and Hogan, D. (2005). *Researching Children's Experience: Approaches and Methods*. London, UK: Sage.

Gregory, A. (2000). 'Problematizing participation: a critical review of approaches to participation in evaluation theory'. *Evaluation: The International Journal of Theory, Research and Practice*, 16 (2), 179–199.

Griffen, V. (1987). *Women, Development and Empowerment: A Pacific Feminist Perspective*. Kuala Lumpur, Malaysia: Asian and Pacific Development Centre.

Griffin, C., Bengry-Howell, A., Hackley, C. Mistral, W. and Szmigin, I. (2009). ' "Every time I do it I absolutely annihilate myself": loss of (self-)consciousness and loss of memory in young people's drinking narratives'. *Sociology*, 43 (3), 457–476.

Groes-Green, C. (2009). 'Health discourse, sexual slang and ideological contradictions among Mozambican youth: implications for method'. *Culture, Health and Sexuality*, 11 (6), 655–668.

———. (2012). 'Ambivalent participation: sex, power, and the anthropologist in Mozambique'. *Medical Anthropology*, 31 (1), 44–60.

Guta, A., Flicker, S. and Roche, B. (2013). 'Governing through community allegiance: a qualitative examination of peer research in community-based participatory research.' *Critical Public Health*, doi:10.1080/09581596.2012.761675.

Habermas, J. (1970). 'Toward a theory of communicative competence'. *Inquiry*, 13 (1–4), 360–375.

———. (1972). *Knowledge and Human Interests*. [Trans. J. Viertel]. London, UK: Heinemann.

Haenfler, R. (2006). *Straight Edge: Clean-Living Youth, Hardcore Punk and Social Change*. New Brunswick, NJ: Rutgers University Press.

Hage, A. and Lorensen, M. (2005). 'A philosophical analysis of the concept of empowerment: the fundament of an education programme to the frail elderly'. *Nursing Philosophy*, 6 (4), 235–246.

Hagquist, C. and Starrin, B. (1997). 'Health education in schools – from information to empowerment models'. *Health Promotion International*, 12 (3), 225–232.

Haines, R. J., Johnson, J. L., Carter, C. I. and Arora, K. (2009). ' "I couldn't say, I'm not a girl" – Adolescents talk about gender and marijuana use'. *Social Science and Medicine*, 68 (11), 2029–2036.

Haines, R. J., Poland, B. D. and Johnson, J. L. (2009). 'Becoming a "real" smoker: cultural capital in young women's accounts of smoking and other substance use'. *Sociology of Health and Illness*, 31 (1), 66–80.

Hall, G. S. (1904). *Adolescence: Its Psychology and its Relation to Physiology, Anthropology, Sociology, Sex, Crime, Religion and Education.* (vol. I). Englewood Cliffs, NJ: Prentice-Hall.

Hall, S. and Jefferson, T. (eds.) (1976). *Resistance Through Rituals: Youth Subcultures in Post-War Britain.* London, UK: Hutchinson.

Hammersley, M. (1987). 'Some notes on the terms "validity" and "reliability" '. *British Educational Research Journal*, 13 (1), 73–81.

———. (2006). 'Ethnography: problems and prospects'. *Ethnography and Education*, 1 (1), 3–14.

Harcourt, D. and Conroy, H. (2005). 'Informed assent: ethics and processes when researching with young children'. *Early Child Development and Care*, 175 (6), 567–577.

Harden, J., Scott, S., Backett-Milburn, K. and Jackson, S. (2000). 'Can't talk, won't talk?: methodological issues in researching children'. *Sociological Research Online*, 5 (2). [Online] Available at: http://www.socresonline.org.uk/5/2/harden.html [Last accessed 18th April 2013].

Harrison, L., Kelly, P., Lindsay, J., Advocat, J. and Hickey, C. (2011). ' "I don't know anyone that has two drinks a day": young people, alcohol and the government of pleasure'. *Health, Risk and Society*, 13 (5), 469–486.

Harstock, N. (1983). *Money, Sex and Power: Toward a Feminist Historical Materialism.* Boston, MA: Northeastern University Press.

Hart, R. (1997). *Children's Participation: The Theory and Practice of Involving Young Citizens in Community Development and Environmental Care.* London, UK: Earthscan.

Harvey, L. and Gill, R. (2011). 'Spicing it up: sexual entrepreneurs and *The Sex Inspectors*'. In R. Gill and C. Scharff (eds.). *New Femininities: Postfeminism, Neoliberalism and Subjectivity.* Basingstoke, UK: Palgrave Macmillan. pp. 52–68.

Hawton, K., Rodham, K., Evans, E. and Weatherall, R. (2002).'Deliberate self-harm in adolescence: self-report survey in schools in England'. *British Medical Journal*, 325 (7374), 1207–1211.

Hearn, J. (2012). *Theorizing Power.* Basingstoke, UK: Hampshire.

Helve, H. and Wallace, C. (2001). *Youth, Citizenship and Empowerment.* Aldershot, UK: Ashgate.

Hennessy, E. and Heary, C. (2005). 'Exploring children's views through focus groups'. In S. Greene and D. Hogan (eds.). *Researching Children's Experience: Approaches and Methods.* London, UK: Sage. pp. 236–253.

Henwood, F., Wyatt, S., Hart, A. and Smith, J. (2003). ' "Ignorance is bliss sometimes": constraints on the emergence of the "informed patient" in the changing landscapes of health information'. *Sociology of Health and Illness*, 25 (6), 589–607.

Hill, M. (2005). 'Ethical considerations in researching children's experiences'. In S. Greene and D. Hogan (eds.). *Researching Children's Experiences*. London, UK: Sage. pp. 61–87.

Hill, M. (2006). 'Children's voices on ways of having a voice: children's and young people's perspectives on methods used in research and consultation'. *Childhood*, 13 (1), 69–89.

Hine, J., Lemetti, F. and Trikha, S. (2004). *Citizenship: Young People's Perspectives*. [Online] Available at: http://dera.ioe.ac.uk/8466/1/dpr10.pdf [Last accessed 18th April 2013].

Hodkinson, P. (2005). 'Insider research in the study of youth cultures'. *Journal of Youth Studies*, 8 (2), 131–149.

Holland, J. (2007). 'Emotions and research'. *International Journal of Social Research Methodology*, 10 (3), 195–209.

Holland, J., Ramazanoglu, C., Sharpe, S. and Thomson, R. (2004). *The Male in the Head: Young People, Heterosexuality and Power*. (2nd ed.). London, UK: Tufnell Press.

Holliday, A. (2007). *Doing and Writing Qualitative Research*. (2nd ed.). London, UK: Sage.

Hollingworth, S. and Williams, K. (2009). 'Constructions of the working-class "Other" among urban, white, middle-class youth: "chavs", subculture and the valuing of education'. *Journal of Youth Studies*, 12 (5), 467–482.

Hoppe, M. J., Graham, L., Wilsdon, A., Wells, E. A., Nahom, D. and Morrison, D. (2004). 'Teens speak out about HIV/AIDS: focus group discussions about risk and decision-making'. *Journal of Adolescent Health*, 35 (2), 27–35.

Horowitz, J. A., Vessey, J. A., Carlson, K. L., Bradley, J. F., Montoya, C. and Mc-Cullough, B. (2003). 'Conducting school-based focus groups: lessons learned from the CATS project'. *Journal of Paediatric Nursing*, 18 (5), 321–331.

Howe, D. (1994). 'Modernity, post-modernity and social work'. *British Journal of Social Work*, 24 (5), 513–532.

Hui, A. and Stickley, T. (2007). 'Mental health policy and mental health service user perspectives on involvement: a discourse analysis'. *Journal of Advanced Nursing*, 59 (4), 416–426.

Humphreys, L. (1975). *Tearoom Trade: Impersonal Sex in Public Places*. New York, NY: Aldine.

Hunt, G. P., Evans, K. and Kares, F. (2007). 'Drug use and meanings of risk and pleasure'. *Journal of Youth Studies*, 10 (1), 73–96.

Hyde, A., Howlett, E., Brady, D. and Drennan, J. (2005). 'The focus group method: insights from focus group interviews on sexual health with adolescents'. *Social Science and Medicine*, 61 (12), 2588–2599.

Ingham, R. (2005). ' "We didn't cover that at school": education *against* pleasure or education *for* pleasure?' *Sex Education: Sexuality, Society and Learning*, 5 (4), 375–388.

———. (2006). 'The importance of context in understanding and seeking to promote sexual health'. In R. Ingham and P. Aggleton (eds.). *Promoting Young People's Sexual Health: International Perspectives*. Abingdon, UK: Routledge. pp. 41–61.

Ioannou, S. (2003). 'Young people's accounts of smoking, exercising, eating and drinking alcohol: being cool or being unhealthy?' *Critical Public Health*, 13 (4), 357–371.

————. (2009). ' "Eating beans . . . that is a 'no-no' for our times": young Cypriots' consumer meanings of "healthy" and "fast" food'. *Health Education Journal,* 68 (3), 186–195.

Israel, B. A., Checkoway, B., Schultz, A. and Zimmerman, M. (1994). 'Health education and community empowerment: conceptualising and measuring perceptions of individual, organisational and community control'. *Health Education Quarterly,* 21 (2), 149–170.

Jackson, C. (2006). ' "Wild" girls? An exploration of "ladette" cultures in secondary schools'. *Gender and Education,* 18 (4), 339–360.

James, A. and Prout, A. (1997). *Constructing and Reconstructing Childhood: Contemporary Issues in the Sociological Study of Childhood.* London, UK: Falmer Press.

Janis, I. L. (1982). *Groupthink.* (2nd ed.). Boston, MA: Houghton Mifflin.

Järvinen, M. (2012). 'A will to health? Drinking, risk and social class'. *Health, Risk and Society,* 14 (3), 241–256.

Järvinen, M. and Gundelach, P. (2007). 'Teenage drinking, symbolic capital and distinction'. *Journal of Youth Studies,* 10 (1), 55–71.

Jayakody, A., Sinha, S., Curtis, K., Roberts, H. and Viner, R. (2005). *Smoking, Drinking, Drug Use, Mental Health and Sexual Behaviour in Young People in East London: Report for the Teenage Pregnancy Unit.* London, UK: DH/DfES.

Jefferson, T. (1976). 'Cultural responses of the Teds'. In S. Hall and T. Jefferson (eds.). *Resistance Through Rituals: Youth Subcultures in Post-War Britain.* London, UK: Hutchinson. pp. 67–71.

Jenks, C. (2005). *Childhood.* (2nd ed.). Abingdon, UK: Routledge.

Jennings, L. B., Parra-Medina, D. M., Messias, D. K. H. and McLoughlin, K. (2006). 'Toward a critical social theory of youth empowerment'. *Journal of Community Practice,* 14 (1–2), 31–55.

Jingree, T. and Finlay, W. M. L. (2012). ' "It's got so politically correct now": parents' talk about empowering individuals with learning disabilities'. *Sociology of Health and Illness,* 34 (3), 412–428.

Johansson, A., Brunnberg, E. and Eriksson, C. (2007). 'Adolescent girls' and boys' perceptions of mental health'. *Journal of Youth Studies,* 10 (2), 183–202.

Johnny, L. (2006). 'Re-conceptualizing childhood: children's rights and youth participation in schools'. *International Education Journal,* 7 (1), 17–25.

Juelskjær, M. (2008). 'Resisting and committing to schooling: intersections of masculinity and academic position'. *International Journal of Qualitative Studies in Education,* 21 (1), 49–63.

Jupp, E. (2007). 'Participation, local knowledge and empowerment: researching public space with young people'. *Environment and Planning,* 39 (12), 2832–2844.

Karl, M. (1995). *Women and Empowerment: Participation and Decision-Making.* London, UK: Zed Books.

Karmaliani, R., McFarlane, J., Asad, N., Madhanj, F., Hirani, S., Shehzad, S. and Zaidi, A. (2009). 'Applying community-based participatory research methods to improve maternal and child health in Karachi, Pakistan'. *Nursing Outlook,* 57 (4), 204–209.

Katainen, A. (2006). 'Challenging the imperative of health? Smoking and justifications of risk-taking'. *Critical Public Health,* 16 (4), 295–305.

Kelly, P. (2000). 'Youth as an artefact of expertise: problematizing the practice of youth studies in an age of uncertainty'. *Journal of Youth Studies,* 3 (3), 301–315.

————. (2003). 'Growing up as a risky business? Risks, surveillance and the institutionalized mistrust of youth'. *Journal of Youth Studies*, 6 (2), 165–180.

————. (2006). 'The entrepreneurial Self and "youth at-risk": exploring the horizons of identity in the twenty-first century'. *Journal of Youth Studies* 9 (1), 17–32.

Kelly, P. J., Lesser, J., Peralez-Dieckmann, E. and Castilla, M. (2007). 'Community-based violence awareness'. *Issues in Mental Health Nursing*, 28 (3), 241–253.

Kendall, S. (1998). *Health and Empowerment: Research and Practice*. London, UK: Arnold.

Kerrigan, R. A., Fonner, V. A., Stromdhal, S. and Kennedy, C. E. (2013). 'Community empowerment among female sex workers is an effective HIV prevention intervention: a systematic review of the peer-reviewed evidence from low-and middle-income countries'. *AIDS Behaviour*, doi:10.1007/s10461-013-0458-4.

Kirby, P., Layon, C., Cronin, K. and Sinclair, R. (2003). *Building a Culture of Participation: Involving Children and Young People in Policy, Service Planning, Delivery and Education*. [Online] Available at: https://www.education.gov.uk/publications /eOrderingDownload/DfES-0827-2003.pdf.pdf [Last accessed 18th April 2013].

Kitzinger, J. (1994). 'The methodology of focus groups: the importance of interaction between research participants'. *Sociology of Health and Illness* 16 (1), 103–121.

Knight, R., Shoveller, J. A., Oliffe, J. L., Gilbert, M., Frank, B. and Ogilvie, G. (2012). 'Masculinities, "guy talk" and "manning up": a discourse analysis of how young men talk about sexual health'. *Sociology of Health and Illness*, 34 (8), 1246–1261.

Krishnan, S., Subbiah, K., Khanum, S., Chandra, P. S. and Padian, N. S. (2012). 'An intergenerational women's empowerment intervention to mitigate domestic violence: results of a pilot study in Bengaluru, India'. *Violence Against Women*, 18 (3), 346–370.

Krueger, R. A. and Casey, M. A. (2009). *Focus Groups: A Practical Guide for Applied Research*. (4th ed.). Thousand Oaks, CA: Sage.

Kubzansky, L. and Kawachi, I. (2000). 'Affective states and health'. In L. F. Berkman and I. Kawachi (eds.). *Social Epidemiology*. Oxford, UK: Oxford University Press. pp. 213–242.

Kuokkanen, L. and Katajisto, J. (2003). 'Promoting or impeding empowerment? *Journal of Nursing Administration*, 33 (4), 209–215.

Kuokkanen, L. and Leino-Kilpi, H. (2001). 'The qualities of an empowered nurse and the factors involved'. *Journal of Nursing Management*, 9 (5), 273–280.

Kuttab, E. (2010). 'Empowerment as resistance: conceptualising Palestinian women's empowerment'. *Development: Gender and Empowerment*, 53 (2), 247–253.

Labonte, R. (1989). 'Community and professional empowerment'. *Canadian Nurse*, 85 (3), 23–30.

————. (1993). *Health Promotion and Empowerment: Practice Frameworks*. Toronto, Ontario, Canada: Centre for Health Promotion and Participation.

————. (1994). 'Health promotion and empowerment: reflections on professional practice'. *Health Education Quarterly*, 21 (2), 253–268.

————. (1996). *Community Development in the Public Health Sector: The Possibilities of an Empowering Relationship between the State and Civil Society*. PhD Thesis. Toronto, Ontario, Canada: York University.

Landstedt, E., Asplund, K. and Gådin, K. G. (2009). 'Understanding adolescent mental health: the influence of social processes, doing gender and gendered power relations'. *Sociology of Health and Illness*, 31 (7), 962–978.

Langhout, R.D. and Thomas, E. (2010). 'Imagining Participatory Action Research in collaboration with children: an introduction'. *American Journal of Community Psychology*, 46 (1–2), 60–66.

Lansley, A. (2010). *Secretary of State for Health's Speech to the UK Faculty of Public Health Conference – 'A New Approach to Public Health'*. [Online]. Available at: http://webarchive.nationalarchives.gov.uk/+/www.dh.gov.uk/en/MediaCentre/Speeches/DH_117280 [Last accessed 18th April 2013].

Latter, S. (1998). 'Health promotion in the acute sector: the case for empowering nurse'. In S. Kendall (ed.). *Health and Empowerment*. London, UK: Arnold , 11–38.

Laverack, G. (2001). 'An identification and interpretation of the organizational aspects of community empowerment'. *Community Development Journal*, 36 (2), 40–52.

———. (2004). *Health Promotion Practice: Power and Empowerment*. London, UK: Sage.

———. (2007). *Health Promotion Practice: Building Empowered Communities*. Maidenhead, UK: Open University Press.

———. (2009). *Public Health: Power, Empowerment and Professional Practice*. (2nd ed.). Basingstoke, UK: Palgrave Macmillan.

Laverack, G. and Wallerstein, N. (2001). 'Measuring community empowerment: a fresh look at organisational domains'. *Health Promotion International*, 16 (2), 179–185.

Laverack, G. and Whipple, A. (2010). 'The sirens' song of empowerment: a case study of health promotion and the New Zealand prostitutes collective'. *Global Health Promotion*, 17 (1), 33–38.

Lazar, M.M. (2011). 'The right to be beautiful: postfeminist identity and consumer beauty advertising'. In R. Gill and C. Scharff (eds.). *New Femininities: Postfeminism, Neoliberalism and Subjectivity*. Basingstoke, UK: Palgrave Macmillan. pp. 37–52.

Lee, M. and Koh, J. (2001). 'Is empowerment really a new concept?' *International Journal of Human Resource Management*, 12 (4), 684–695.

Lee, N. (2001). *Childhood and Society: Growing Up in an Age of Uncertainty*. Maidenhead, UK: Open University Press.

Lewis, A. and Lindsay, G. (2000). *Researching Children's Perspectives*. Buckingham, UK: Open University Press.

Lincoln, N.D., Travers, C., Ackers, P. and Wilkinson, A. (2002). 'The meaning of empowerment: the interdisciplinary etymology of a new management concept'. *International Journal of Management Reviews*, 4 (3), 271–290.

Lindsay, J. (2009). 'Young Australians and the staging of intoxication and self-control'. *Journal of Youth Studies*, 12 (4), 371–384.

Lovell, T. (2003). 'Resisting with authority: historical specificity, agency and the performative self'. *Theory, Culture and Society*, 20 (1), 1–17.

Lukes, S. (1974). *Power: A Radical View*. Basingstoke, UK: Palgrave Macmillan.

———. (2005). *Power: A Radical View*. (2nd ed.). Basingstoke, UK: Palgrave Macmillan.

Lupton, D. (1994). *Medicine as Culture*. London, UK: Sage.

———. (1995). *The Imperative of Health: Public Health and the Regulated Body*. London, UK: Sage.

———. (1999a). *Risk*. London, UK: Routledge.

————. (1999b). *Risk and Sociocultural Theory: New Directions and Perspectives.* Cambridge, UK: Cambridge University Press.

————. (2005). 'Lay discourses and beliefs related to food risks: an Australian perspective'. *Sociology of Health and Illness,* 27 (4), 448–467.

————. (2013). *Fat.* Abingdon, UK: Routledge

Lupton, D. and Tulloch, J. (2002). 'Life would be pretty dull without risk: voluntary risk-taking and its pleasures'. *Health, Risk and Society,* 4 (2), 113–124.

Macedo, S. (1995). 'Multiculturalism for the religious right? Defending liberal civic education'. *Journal of Philosophy of Education,* 29 (2), 223–238.

Machiavelli, N. (1958). *The Prince.* [Trans. W. Marriott]. London, UK: Macmillan. [Original work published 1517].

Mackinnon, C. (1987). *Feminism Unmodified: Discourses on Life and Law.* Cambridge, MA: Harvard University Press.

Macvarish, J. (2010). 'The effect of "risk-thinking" on the contemporary construction of teenage motherhood'. *Health, Risk and Society,* 12 (4), 313–322.

Maes, L. and Lievens, J. (2003). 'Can the school make a difference? A multilevel analysis of adolescent risk and health behaviour'. *Social Science and Medicine,* 56 (3), 517–529.

Mallan, K.M., Singh, P. and Giardina, N. (2010). 'The challenges of participatory research with 'tech-savvy' youth'. *Journal of Youth Studies,* 13 (2), 255–272.

Mannheim, K. (1952). *Essays on the Sociology of Knowledge.* London, UK: Routledge and Kegan Paul.

Mannion, G. (2007). 'Going spatial, going relational: why 'listening to children' and children's participation needs reframing'. *Discourse,* 28 (3), 405–420.

Manojlovich, M. (2007). 'Power and empowerment in nursing: looking backward to inform the future'. *The Online Journal of Issues in Nursing,* 12 (1), 1–16.

Marston, C., King, E. and Ingham, R. (2006). 'Young people and condom use: findings from qualitative research'. In R. Ingham and P. Aggleton (eds.). *Promoting Young People's Sexual Health: International Perspectives.* Abingdon, UK: Routledge. pp. 27–41.

Martin, G.P. and Finn, R. (2011). 'Patients as team members: opportunities, challenges and paradoxes of including patients in multi-professional healthcare teams'. *Sociology of Health and Illness,* 33 (7), 1050–1065.

Marx, K. and Engels, F. (1959). 'Excerpts from *The German Ideology*'. In L. Feller (ed.). *Marx and Engels: Basic Writings on Politics and Philosophy.* Glasgow, UK: William Collins, 287–302.

Mason, J. and Fallon, J. (2001). 'Some Sydney children define abuse: implications for agency in childhood'. In L. Alanen and B. Mayall (eds.). *Conceptualizing Child–Adult Relations.* London, UK: Routledge Falmer. pp. 99–114.

Masson, J. (2000). 'Researching children's perspectives: legal issues'. In A. Lewis and G. Lindsay (eds.). *Researching Children's Perspectives.* Buckingham, UK: Open University Press. pp. 34–46.

Mauthner, M. (1997). 'Methodological aspects of collecting data from children: lessons learnt from three research projects'. *Children and Society,* 11 (1), 16–28.

Mayall, B. (1994). *Negotiating Health.* London, UK: Cassell.

————. (1996). *Children, Health and the Social Order.* Buckingham, UK: Open University Press.

————. (2002). *Towards a Sociology for Childhood: Thinking from Children's Lives.* Buckingham, UK: Open University Press.

McCarry, M. (2012). 'Who benefits? A critical reflection of children and young people's participation in sensitive research'. *International Journal of Social Research Methodology*, 15 (1), 55–68.

McDaid, S. (2010). 'Redefining empowerment in mental health: an analysis using Hannah Arendt's power concept'. *Journal of Power*, 3 (2), 209–225.

McGee, R. and Williams, S. (2000). 'Does low self-esteem predict health compromising behaviours among adolescents?' *Journal of Adolescence*, 23 (5), 569–582.

McLafferty, I. (2004). 'Focus group interviews as a data collection strategy'. *Journal of Advanced Nursing* 48 (2), 187–194.

McNay, L. (2000). *Gender and Agency: Reconfiguring the Subject in Feminist and Social Theory*. Cambridge, UK: Polity.

———. (2003). 'Agency, anticipation and indeterminacy in feminist theory'. *Feminist Theory*, 4 (2), 139–148.

McRobbie, A. (1978). 'Working class girls and the culture of femininity'. In Women's Studies Group, Centre for Contemporary Cultural Studies (eds.). *Women Take Issue: Aspects of Women's Subordination*. London, UK: Hutchinson. pp. 96–108.

Messias, D. K. H., Jennings, L. B., Fore, M. E., McLoughlin, K. and Parra-Medina, D. (2008). 'Societal images of youth: representations and interpretations of youth actively engaged in their communities'. *International Journal of Qualitative Studies in Education*, 21 (2), 159–178.

Meyrick, J. (2005). 'Approval procedures and passive consent considerations in research among young people'. *Health Education*, 105 (4), 249–258.

Milbourne, L. (2009). 'Valuing difference or securing compliance? Working to involve young people in community settings'. *Children and Society*, 23 (5), 347–363.

Miliband, R. (1969). *The State in Capitalist Society*. London, UK: Quartet.

Milio, N. (1986). *Promoting Health through Public Policy*. Ottawa, Ontario, Canada: Canadian Public Health Association.

Mill, J. S. (1970). 'The subjection of women'. In A. Rossi (ed.). *Essays on Sex Equality*. Chicago, IL: University of Chicago Press. pp. 123–242.

Milstein, D. (2010). 'Children as co-researchers in anthropological narratives in education'. *Ethnography and Education*, 5 (1), 1–15.

Minkler, M. (1985). 'Building supportive ties and sense of community among the inner-city elderly: the Tenderloin Senior Outreach Project'. *Health Education and Behaviour*, 12 (4), 303–314.

Mitchell, L. (1997). 'Pressure groups: young people's accounts of peer pressure to smoke'. *Social Sciences in Health*, 3 (1), 3–17.

Mitchell, W. A., Crawshaw, P., Bunton, R. and Green, E. E. (2001). 'Situating young people's experiences of risk and identity'. *Health, Risk and Society*, 3 (2), 217–233.

Mohajer, N. and Earnest, J. (2009). 'Youth empowerment for the most vulnerable: A model based on the pedagogy of Freire and experiences in the field'. *Health Education*, 109 (5), 424–438.

———. (2010). 'The challenge of low literacy in health promotion: using empowerment methods with out-of-school adolescents in North India'. *Vulnerable Children and Youth Studies*, 5 (1), 88–96.

Monaghan, L. F. and Malson, H. (2013). "It's worse for women and girls': negotiating embodied masculinities through weight-related talk'. *Critical Public Health*, doi: 10.1080/09581596.2012.754843.

Morgan, A. and Ziglio, E. (2007). 'Revitalizing the evidence base for public health: an assets model'. *Promotion and Education*, 14 (suppl. 2): 17–22.

Morgan, M. (2007). 'Hospitals and patient care'. In G. Scrambler (ed.). *Sociology as Applied to Medicine.* (6th ed.). London, UK: Saunders. pp. 71–83.

Morrow, V.M. (2000). '"Dirty looks" and "trampy places" in young people's accounts of community and neighbourhood: implications for health inequalities'. *Critical Public Health,* 10 (2), 141–152.

Morrow, V.M. (2001). 'Using qualitative methods to elicit young people's perspectives on their environments: some ideas for community health initiatives'. *Health Education Research,* 16 (3), 255–268.

Morrow, V. and Mayall, B. (2009). 'What is wrong with children's well-being in the UK? Questions of meaning and measurement'. *Journal of Social Welfare & Family Law,* 31 (3), 217–229.

Morton, M. and Montgomery, P. (2011). *Youth Empowerment Programs for Improving Self-efficacy and Self-esteem of Adolescents.* Campbell Systematic Reviews. doi:10.4073/csr.2011.5.

Mosedale, S. (2005). 'Assessing women's empowerment: towards a conceptual framework'. *Journal of International Development,* 7 (2), 243–257.

Moss, B. (2005). *Religion and Spirituality.* Lyme Regis, UK: Russell House.

Naidoo, J. and Wills, J. (2009). *Health Promotion: Foundations for Practice.* (3rd ed.). London, UK: Baillière Tindall.

Nation, M., Vieno, A., Perkins, D.D. and Santinello, M. (2008). 'Bullying in school and adolescent sense of empowerment: an analysis of relationships with parents, friends and teachers'. *Journal of Community and Applied Social Psychology,* 18 (3), 211–232.

Nelson, A.L., MacDonald, D. and Abbott, R.A. (2012). 'A risky business? Health and physical activity from the perspectives of urban Australian Indigenous young people'. *Health, Risk and Society,* 14 (4), 325–340.

Nichter, M., Nichter, M., Lloyd-Richardson, E., Flaherty, B., Carkoglu, A. and Taylor, N. (2006). 'Gendered dimensions of smoking among college students'. *Journal of Adolescent Research,* 21 (3), 215–243.

Ning, S., Zhong, H., Libo, W. and Qiujie, L. (2009). 'The impact of nurse empowerment on job satisfaction'. *Journal of Advanced Nursing,* 65 (12), 2642–2648.

Office for National Statistics [ONS] (2011). *Neighbourhood Statistics.* [Online]. Available at: http://www.neighbourhood.statistics.gov.uk/dissemination/ [Last accessed 18th April 2013].

Okin, S.M. (1989). *Justice, Gender and the Family.* New York, NY: Basic Books.

Oliffe, J.L., Chabot, C., Knight, R., Davis, W., Bungay, V. and Shoveller, J.A. (2013). 'Women on men's sexual health and sexually transmitted infection testing: a gender relations analysis'. *Sociology of Health and Illness,* 35 (1), 1–16.

Parsons, T. (1967). *Sociological Theory and Modern Society.* New York, NY: Free Press.

Pascoe, C.J. (2007). *Dude, you're a Fag: Masculinity and Sexuality in High School.* Berkeley: University of California Press.

Pearrow, M.M. and Pollack, S. (2009). 'Youth empowerment in oppressive systems: opportunities for school consultants'. *Journal of Educational and Psychological Consultation,* 19 (1), 45–60.

Pearson, J. (2006). 'Personal control, self-efficacy in sexual negotiation, and contraceptive risk among adolescents: the role of gender'. *Sex Roles,* 54 (9–10), 615–625.

Pease, B. (2002). 'Rethinking empowerment: a postmodern reappraisal for emancipatory practice'. *British Journal of Social Work,* 32 (2), 135–147.

Percy-Smith, B. (2006). 'From consultation to social learning in community participation with young people'. *Children, Youth and Environments,* 16 (2), 153–179.
———. (2007). ' "You think you know? . . . you have no idea": youth participation in health policy development'. *Health Education Research,* 22 (6), 879–894.
Percy-Smith, B. and Thomas, N. (eds.) (2010). A *Handbook of Children and Young People's Participation: Perspectives from Theory & Practice.* Abingdon, UK: Routledge.
Perrons, D. and Skyers, S. (2003). 'Empowerment through participation? Conceptual explorations and a case study'. *International Journal of Urban and Regional Research,* 27 (2), 265–285.
Peterson, Z. (2010). 'What is sexual empowerment? A multidimensional and process-orientated approach to adolescent girls' sexual empowerment'. *Sex Roles,* 62 (5–6): 307–313.
Pilcher, J. (1994). 'Mannheim's sociology of generations: an undervalued legacy'. *British Journal of Sociology,* 45 (3), 481–495.
Pilkington, H. (2007). 'In good company: risk, security and choice in young people's drug decisions'. *The Sociological Review,* 55 (2), 373–392.
Pinkey, S. (2011). 'Participation and emotions: troubling encounters between children and social welfare professionals'. *Children and Society,* 25 (1), 37–46.
Porter, S. (1992). 'The poverty of professionalization: a critical analysis of strategies for the occupational advancement of nursing'. *Journal of Advanced Nursing,* 17 (6), 720–726.
Poulantzas, N. (1976). *State, Power, Socialism.* London, UK: New Left Books.
Poulton, B. (1999). 'User involvement in identifying health needs and shaping and evaluating services: is it being realised?' *Journal of Advanced Nursing,* 30 (6), 1289–1296.
Prins, E. (2008). 'Adult literacy education, gender equity and empowerment: insights from a Freirean-inspired literacy programme'. *Studies in the Education of Adults,* 40 (1), 24–39.
Prochaska, J.O. and DiClimente, C.C. (1984). *The Trans-theoretical Approach: Crossing Traditional Boundaries of Therapy.* Homewood, IL: Dow Jones Irwin.
Punch, S. (2002a). 'Research with children: the same or different from research with adults?' *Childhood,* 9 (3), 321–341.
———. (2002b). 'Interviewing strategies with young people: the "secret box", stimulus material and task-based activities'. *Children and Society,* 16 (1), 45–56.
Putnam, R. (1993). 'The prosperous community: social capital and public life'. *American Prospect,* 4 (13), 35–42.
———. (1995). 'Bowling alone: America's declining social capital'. *Journal of Democracy,* 6 (1), 65–79.
Qvortrup, J., Corsaro, W.A. and Honig, M.-S. (eds.) (2009). *The Palgrave Handbook of Childhood Studies.* Basingstoke, UK: Macmillan.
Raby, R. (2002). 'A tangle of discourses: teenage girls negotiating identity'. *Journal of Youth Studies,* 5 (4), 425–450.
———. (2005). 'What is resistance?' *Journal of Youth Studies,* 8 (2), 151–171.
———. (2010). ' "Tank tops are OK but I don't want to see her thong": Girls' engagements with secondary school dress codes'. *Youth and Society,* 41 (3), 333–356.
Rappaport, J. (1984). 'Studies in empowerment: introduction to the issue'. *Prevention in Human Sciences,* 3 (1), 1–7.

Rees, R., Oliver, K., Woodman, J. and Thomas, J. (2011). 'The views of young children in the UK about obesity, body size, shape and weight: a systematic review'. *BMC Public Health*, 11, 188–199.

Reininger, B., Evans, A. E., Griffin, S. F., Valois, R. F., Vincent, M. L., Parra-Medina, D., Taylor, D. J. and Zullig, K. J. (2003). 'Development of a youth survey to measure risk behaviours, attitudes and assets: examining multiple influences'. *Health Education Research*, 18 (4), 461–476.

Renold, E. (2004). 'Other boys: negotiating non-hegemonic masculinities in the primary school'. *Gender and Education*, 16 (2), 248–266.

Respect Task Force. (2006). *Respect Action Plan*. London, UK: Home Office.

Rex, J. (1971). 'Typology and objectivity: a comment on Weber's four sociological methods'. In A. Sahay (ed.). *Max Weber and Modern Sociology*. London, UK: Routledge and Kegan Paul. pp. 17–37.

———. (1974). *Sociology and the Demystification of the Modern World*. London, UK: Routledge and Kegan Paul.

Richman, L. S., Kubzansky, L. K., Maselko, J., Kawachi, I., Choo, P. and Bauer, M. (2005). 'Positive emotion and health: going beyond the negative'. *Health Psychology*, 24 (4), 422–429.

Ridder, M. A.M., Heuvelmans, M. A., Visscher, T. L. S., Seidell, J. C. and Renders, C. M. (2010). ' "We are healthy so we can behave unhealthily": a qualitative study of the health behaviour of Dutch lower vocational students'. *Health Education*, 110 (1), 30–42.

Rifkin, S. (1990). *Community Participation in Maternal and Child Health/Family Planning Programmes*. Geneva, Switzerland: WHO.

Rindner, E. C. (2002). 'Using Freirian empowerment for health education with adolescents in primary, secondary and tertiary psychiatric settings'. *Journal of Child Psychiatric Nursing*, 17 (2), 78–85.

Rissel, C. (1994). 'Empowerment: the holy grail of health promotion?' *Health Promotion International*, 9 (1), 39–47.

Robinson, C. and Kellett, M. (2004). 'Power'. In S. Fraser, V. Lewis, S. Ding, M. Kellett and C. Robinson (eds.). *Doing Research with Children and Young People*. London, UK: Sage. pp. 81–97.

Robson, C. (2011). *Real World Research*. (3rd ed.). Chichester, UK: Wiley.

Rodwell, C. M. (1996). 'An analysis of the concept of empowerment'. *Journal of Advanced Nursing*, 23 (2), 305–313.

Romero, L., Wallerstein, N., Lucero, J., Fredine, H. G., Keefe, J. and O'Connell, J. (2006). 'Woman to woman: coming together for positive change – using empowerment and popular education to prevent HIV in women'. *AIDS Education and Prevention*, 18 (5), 390–405.

Room, R. and Sato, H. (2002). 'Drinking and drug use in youth cultures: building identity and community'. *Contemporary Drug Problems*, 29 (1), 5–12.

Rotter, J. (1966). 'Generalized expectations for internal versus external control of reinforcement'. *Psychological Monographs*, 80 (1), 1–28.

Rowlands, J. (1998). 'A word of the times, but what does it mean? Empowerment in the discourse and practice of development'. In H. Afshar (ed.). *Women and Empowerment: Illustrations from the Third World*. Basingstoke, UK: Palgrave Macmillan. pp. 11–34.

Rowling, L. (2009). 'Strengthening "school" in school mental health promotion'. *Health Education*, 109 (4), 357–368.

Rugkåsa, J., Stewart-Knox, B., Sittlington, J., Abaunza, P. S. and Treacy, M. P. (2003). 'Hard boys, attractive girls: expressions of gender in young people's conversations on smoking in Northern Ireland'. *Health Promotion International*, 18 (4), 307–314.

Ruston, A. (2009). 'Isolation: a threat and means of spatial control. Living with risk in a deprived neighbourhood'. *Health, Risk and Society*, 11 (3), 257–268.

Rütten, A. and Gelius, P. (2011). 'The interplay of structure and agency in health promotion: integrating a concept of structural change and the policy dimension into a multi-level model and applying it to health promotion principles and practice'. *Social Science and Medicine*, 73 (7), 953–959.

Ryles, S. M. (1999). 'A concept analysis of empowerment: its relationship to mental health nursing'. *Journal of Advanced Nursing*, 29 (3), 600–607.

Salovey, P., Rothman, A. J., Detweiler, J. B. and Steward, W. T. (2000). 'Emotional states and physical health'. *American Psychologist*, 55 (1), 110–121.

Salvage, J. (1992). 'The new nursing: empowering patients or empowering nurses?' In J. Robinson, A. Gray and R. Elkan (ed.). *Policy Issues in Nursing*. Milton Keynes, UK: Open University Press. pp. 9–23.

Sardenberg, C. M. B. (2010). 'Women's empowerment in Brazil: tensions in discourse and practice'. *Development: Gender and Empowerment*, 53 (2), 232–238.

Scadding, J. G. (1988). 'Health and disease: what can medicine do for philosophy?' *Journal of Medical Ethics*, 14 (3), 118–124.

Schulz, A. J., Israel, B. A., Zimmerman, M. A. and Checkoway, B. N. (1995). 'Empowerment as a multi-level construct: perceived control at the individual, organisational and community levels'. *Health Education Research*, 10 (3), 309–327.

Schütz, A. (1963a). 'Common-sense and scientific interpretation of human action'. In M. A. Natanson (ed.). *Philosophy of the Social Sciences*, New York, NY: Random House. pp. 302–346.

———. (1963b). 'Concept and theory formation in the social sciences'. In M. A. Natanson (ed.). *Philosophy of the Social Sciences*. New York, NY: Random House. pp. 231–249.

Scott, J. C. (1990). *Domination and the Arts of Resistance: Hidden Transcripts*. New Haven, CT: Yale University Press.

Scriven, A. and Stiddard, L. (2003). 'Empowering schools: translating health promotion principles into practice'. *Health Education*, 103 (2), 110–118.

Seedhouse, D. (2001). *Health: The Foundations for Achievement*. (2nd ed.). Chichester, UK: Wiley.

Shearer, C., Hosterman, S. J., Gillen, M. M. and Lefkowitz, E. S. (2005). 'Are traditional gender role attitudes associated with risky sexual behaviour and condom-related beliefs?' *Sex Roles*, 52 (5–6), 311–324.

Shepherd, J., Kavanagh, J., Picot, J., Cooper, K., Harden, A., Barnett-Page, E., Jones, J., Clegg, A., Hartwell, D., Frampton, G. K. and Price, A. (2010). 'The effectiveness and cost-effectiveness of behavioural interventions for the prevention of sexually transmitted infections for young people aged 13–19 years: a systematic review and economic evaluation'. *Health Technology Assessment*, 14 (7), 1–206.

Shoveller, J. A., Johnson, J. L., Langille, D. B. and Mitchell, T. (2004). 'Socio-cultural influences on young people's sexual development'. *Social Science and Medicine*, 59 (3), 473–487.

Shoveller, J. A., Knight, R. E., Johnson, J. L., Oliffe, J. L. and Goldenberg, S. (2010). ' "Not the swab!" Young men's experiences with STI testing'. *Sociology of Health and Illness*, 32 (1), 57–73.

Sixsmith, J., Gabhainn, S. N., Fleming, C. and O'Higgins, S. (2007). 'Children's, parents' and teachers' perceptions of child wellbeing'. *Health Education*, 107 (6), 511–523.

Skelton, R. (1994). 'Nursing and empowerment: concepts and strategies'. *Journal of Advanced Nursing*, 19 (3), 415–423.

Skidmore, D. and Hayter, E. (2000). 'Risk and sex: ego-centricity and sexual behaviour in young adults'. *Health, Risk and Society*, 2 (1), 23–32.

Skidmore, P., Bound, K., and Lownsbrough, H. (2006). *Community Participation: Who Benefits?* London, UK: Joseph Rowntree Foundation.

Smith, A., Martin, S. and the McCreary Centre Society (2010). *Measuring Our Health: Domains and Indicators of Youth Health & Well-Being in British Columbia – Youth's Feedback and Suggestions*. Vancouver, British Columbia, Canada: McCreary Centre Society.

Smith, R., Monaghan, M. and Broad, B. (2003). 'Involving young people as co-researchers: facing up to the methodological issues'. *Qualitative Social Work*, 1 (2), 191–207.

Soto, L. D. and Swadener, B. B. (2005). *Power and Voice in Research with Children*. New York, NY: Peter Lang.

Spencer, G. (2008). 'Young people's perspectives on health-related risks'. *Educate~*, 8 (1), 15–28.

———. (2011). *Empowerment, Young People and Health*. Unpublished PhD thesis, Institute of Education, University of London.

———. (2013a). 'Young people and health: towards a conceptual framework for understanding empowerment'. *Health*, doi:10.1177/1363459312473616.

———. (2013b). 'Young people's perspectives on health: empowerment, or risk?' *Health Education*, 113 (2), 115–131.

———. (2013c). 'The "healthy" self and "risky" young Other: Young people's interpretations of health and health-risks.' *Health, Risk and Society*. doi.org/10.1080/13698575.2013.804037.

Spencer, G., Doull, M. & Shoveller, J. A. (2012). 'Examining the concept of choice in sexual health interventions for young people'. *Youth and Society*, doi:10.1177/0044118X12451277.

Spencer, G., Maxwell, C., & Aggleton, P. (2008). 'What does empowerment mean in school-based Sex and Relationship Education?' *Sex Education: Sexuality, Society and Learning*, 8 (3), 345–356.

Ssewamala, F. M., Sperber, E., Blake, C. A. and Ilic, V. P. (2012). 'Increasing opportunities for inner-city youth: the feasibility of an economic empowerment model in East Harlem and the South Bronx'. *Child and Youth Services Review*, 34 (1), 218–224.

Stanley, N. (2005). 'Thrills and spills: young people's sexual behavior and attitudes in seaside and rural areas'. *Health, Risk and Society*, 7 (4), 337–348.

Starkey, F. (2003). 'The "empowerment debate": consumerist, professional and liberational perspectives in health and social care'. *Social Policy and Society*, 2 (4), 273–284.

Stead, M., McDermott, L. MacKintosh, A. M. and Adamson, A. (2011). 'Why healthy eating is bad for young people's health: identity, belonging and food'. *Social Science and Medicine*, 72 (7), 1131–1139.

Stjerna, M-L., Lauritzen, S. O. and Tillgren, P. (2004). ' "Social thinking" and cultural images: teenagers' notions of tobacco use'. *Social Science and Medicine*, 59 (3), 573–583.

Stone, N. and Ingham, R. (2002). 'Factors affecting British teenagers' contraceptive use at first intercourse: the importance of partner communication'. *Perspectives on Sexual and Reproductive Health*, 34 (4), 191–197.

Story, M., Neumark-Sztainer, and French, S. (2002). 'Individual and environmental influences in adolescents eating behaviours'. *Journal of American Dietary Association*, 102 (3), 40–51.

Stovall, D. (2006). 'Forging community in race and class: critical race theory and the quest for social justice in education'. *Race, Ethnicity and Education*, 9 (3), 243–259.

Sussman, S., Burton, D., Dent, C. W., Stacy, A. W. and Flay, B. R. (1991). 'Use of focus groups in developing an adolescent tobacco use cessation program: collective norm effects'. *Journal of Applied Social Psychology*, 21 (21), 1772–1782.

Swartz, D. L. (2007). 'Recasting power in its third dimensions: review of Steven Lukes' *Power: A Radical Review*'. *Theory and Society*, 36 (1), 103–109.

Tengland, P.-A. (2007). 'Empowerment: A goal or a means for health promotion?' *Medicine, Health Care and Philosophy*, 10 (2), 197–207.

———. (2008). 'Empowerment: A conceptual discussion'. *Health Care Analysis*, 16 (2), 77–96.

Testa, A. C. and Coleman, L. M. (2006). 'Accessing research participants in schools: a case study of a UK adolescent sexual health survey'. *Health Education Research*, 21 (4), 518–526.

Thomas, N. (2007). 'Towards a theory of children's participation'. *International Journal of Children's Rights*, 15 (2), 199–218.

Thompson, L. and Kumar, A. (2011). 'Responses to health promotion campaigns: resistance, denial and othering'. *Critical Public Health*, 21 (1), 105–117.

Thompson, N. (2002). *Building the Future: Social Work with Children, Young People and their Families*. Lyme Regis, UK: Russell House.

Thompson, N. (2007). *Power and Empowerment*. Lyme Regis, UK: Russell House.

Tisdall, K. and Davis, J. (2004). 'Making a difference? Bringing children's and young people's views into policy making'. *Children and Society*, 18 (2), 131–142.

Tolman, D. L. (1999). 'Femininity as a barrier to positive sexual health for adolescent girls'. *Journal of the American Medical Women's Association*, 54 (3), 133–138.

Tones, K. (1998a). 'Empowerment for health: the challenge'. In S. Kendall (ed.). *Health and Empowerment: Research and Practice*. London, UK: Arnold. pp. 185–204.

———. (1998b). 'Health education and the promotion of health: seeking wisely to empower'. In S. Kendall (ed.). *Health and Empowerment: Research and Practice*. London, UK: Arnold. pp. 57–88.

———. (2001). 'Health promotion: the empowerment imperative'. In A. Scriven and J. Orme (eds.). *Health Promotion: Professional Perspectives*. (2nd ed.). Basingstoke, UK: Palgrave. pp. 3–18.

Tones, K. and Tilford, S. (2001). *Health Promotion: Effectiveness, Efficiency and Equity*. (3rd ed.). Cheltenham, UK: Nelson Thornes.

Townsend, P. and Davidson, N. (1982). *Inequalities in Health: The Black Report*. Harmondsworth, UK: Penguin.

Tucker, E. (2007). 'Measurement as a rigorous science: how ethnographic research methods can contribute to the generation and modification of indicators'. In G. Walford (ed.). *Studies in Educational Ethnography: Methodological Developments in Ethnography*. Kidlington, UK: Elsevier. pp. 109–135.

Tucker, F. (2003). 'Sameness or difference? Exploring girls' use of recreational spaces'. *Children's Geographies*, 1 (1), 111–124.

Tulloch, J. and Lupton, D. (2003). *Risk and Everyday Life*. London, UK: Sage.

Turner, K. M. and Gordon, J. (2004). 'A fresh perspective on a rank issue: pupils' accounts of staff enforcement of smoking restrictions'. *Health Education Research*, 19 (2), 148–158.

Tutenges, S. and Rod, M. H. (2009). ' "We got incredibly drunk . . . it was damned fun": drinking stories among Danish youth'. *Journal of Youth Studies*, 12 (4), 355–370.

Ungar, M. and Teram, E. (2000). 'Drifting toward mental health: high-risk adolescents and the process of empowerment'. *Youth and Society*, 32 (2), 228–252.

United Nations [UN] Assembly. (1989). *United Nations Convention on the Rights of the Child (UNCRC) 1989*. Geneva, Switzerland: United Nations.

United Nations Children's Fund [UNICEF]. (2007). *Child Poverty in Perspective – An Overview of Child Well-Being in Rich Countries: A Comprehensive Assessment of the Lives and Well-Being of Children in the Economically Advanced Nations*. Florence, Italy: Innocenti Research Centre.

United Nations Population Fund [UNFPA]. (2006). *Empowering Young Women to Lead Change*. New York, NY: United Nations Population Fund.

Valaitis, R. (2002). ' "They don't trust us; we're just kids" views about community from predominantly female inner city youth'. *Health Care for Women International*, 23 (3), 248–266.

van Exel, N. J. A., de Graaf, G. and Brouwer, W. B. F. (2006). ' "Everyone dies, so you might as well have fun!" Attitudes of Dutch youths about their health and lifestyle'. *Social Science and Medicine*, 63 (10), 2628–2639.

Walford, G. (2007). *Studies in Educational Ethnography: Methodological Developments in Ethnography*. Kidlington, UK: Elsevier.

———. (2008). 'The nature of educational ethnography'. In G. Walford (ed.). *How to do Educational Ethnography*. London, UK: Tufnell Press. pp. 1–15.

Walkerdine, V., Lucey, H., and Melody, J. (2002). 'Subjectivity and qualitative method'. In T. May (ed.). *Qualitative Research in Action*. London, UK: Sage. pp. 179–197.

Wallerstein, N. (2002). 'Empowerment to reduce health disparities'. *Scandinavian Journal of Public Health*, 30 (3), 72–77.

———. (2006). *What is the Evidence on Effectiveness of Empowerment to Improve Health?* Copenhagen, Denmark: WHO Regional Office for Europe.

Wallerstein, N. and Bernstein, E. (1988). 'Empowerment education: Freire's ideas adapted to health education'. *Health Education and Behaviour*, 15 (4), 379–394.

———. (1994). 'Introduction to community empowerment: participatory education and health'. *Health Education Quarterly*, 21 (2), 141–148.

Wallerstein, N. and Sanchez-Merki, V. (1994). 'Freirian praxis in health education: research results from an adolescent prevention program'. *Health Education Research*, 9 (1), 105–118.

Wallerstein, N., Sanchez-Merki, V. and Velarde, L. (2005). 'Freirian praxis in health education and community organizing: a case study of an adolescent prevention program'. In M. Minkler (ed.), *Community Organizing and Community Building for Health*. New Brunswick, NJ: Rutgers University Press. pp. 218–236.

Warwick, I., Aggleton, P., Chase, E., Schagen, S., Blenkinsop, S., Schagen, I., Scott, E. and Eggers, M. (2005). 'Evaluating healthy schools: perceptions of impact among school-based participants'. *Health Education Research*, 20 (6), 697–708.

Watts, J. H. (2011). 'Ethical and practical challenges of participant observation in sensitive health research'. *International Journal of Social Research Methodology,* 14 (4), 301–312.

Webb, T. L. and Sheeran, P. (2006). 'Does changing behavioural intentions engender behaviour change? A meta-analysis of the experimental evidence'. *Psychological Bulletin,* 132 (2), 249–268.

Weber, M. (1947). *The Theory of Social and Economic Organisation.* [Trans. A.M. Henderson and T. Parsons]. New York, NY: Free Press.

Weine, S., Golobof, A., Bahromov, M., Kashuba, A., Kalandarov, T., Jonbekov, J. and Loue, S. (2013). 'Female migrant sex workers in Moscow: gender and power factors and HIV risk'. *Women's Health,* 53 (1), 56–73.

West, P. and Sweeting, H. (1997). ' "Lost souls" and "rebels": a challenge to the assumption that low self-esteem and unhealthy lifestyles are related'. *Health Education,* 97 (5), 161–167.

Westcott, H. L. and Littleton, K. S. (2005). 'Exploring meaning in interviews with children'. In S. Greene and D. Hogan (eds.). *Researching Children's Experience: Approaches and Methods.* London, UK: Sage. pp. 141–158.

Whitehead, M. (1988). *The Health Divide.* London, UK: Routledge.

Whittemore, R., Chase, S. K. and Mandle, C. L. (2001). 'Validity in qualitative research'. *Qualitative Health Research,* 11 (4), 522–537.

Wiggins, N. (2011). 'Popular education for health promotion and community empowerment: a review of the literature'. *Health Promotion International,* 27 (3), 356–371.

Wight, D. and Dixon, H. (2004). '*SHARE* – Sexual Health And Relationships: Safe, Happy And Responsible'. *Education and Health,* 22 (1), 3–7.

Wild, L. G., Flisher, A. J., Bhana, A. and Lombard, C. (2004). 'Associations among adolescent risk behaviours and self-esteem in six domains'. *Journal of Child Psychology and Psychiatry,* 45 (8), 1454–1467.

Wilkinson, R. (1996). *Unhealthy Societies: The Afflictions of Inequality.* London, UK: Routledge.

Williams, G. H. (2003). 'The determinants of health: structure, context and agency'. *Sociology of Health and Illness,* 25 (3), 131–154.

Williams, L. and Labonte, R. (2007). 'Empowerment for migrant communities: paradoxes for practitioners'. *Critical Public Health,* 17 (4), 365–379.

Willis, P. (1977). *Learning to Labour: How Working Class Kids Get Working Class Jobs.* London, UK: Saxon House.

Wills, W. J., Appleton, J. V., Magnusson, J. and Brooks, F. (2008). 'Exploring the limitations of an adult-led agenda for understanding the health behaviours of young people'. *Health and Social Care in the Community,* 16 (3), 244–252.

Wilson, L. (2009). 'Pupil participation: comments from a case study'. *Health Education,* 109 (1), 86–102.

Wilson, N., Minkler, M., Dasho, S., Wallerstein, N. and Martin, A. C. (2008). 'Getting to social action: the Youth Empowerment Strategies (YES!) project'. *Health Promotion Practice,* 9 (4), 395–403.

Woodgate, R. L. and Leach, J. (2010). 'Youth's perspectives on the determinants of health'. *Qualitative Health Research,* 20 (9), 1173–1182.

World Health Organization [WHO]. (1946). *Constitution.* Geneva, Switzerland: WHO.

———. (1977). *Alma Ata Declaration*. Geneva, Switzerland: WHO Regional Office for Europe.

———. (1986). *Ottawa Charter for Health Promotion*. Geneva, Switzerland: WHO Regional Office for Europe.

———. (2005). *The Bangkok Charter for Health Promotion in a Globalized World. 6th Global Conference on Health Promotion*. Bangkok, Thailand: WHO.

———. (2011a). *Making Health Services Adolescent Friendly: Developing National Quality Standards for Adolescent-Friendly Health Services*. Geneva, Switzerland: WHO.

———. (2011b). *Young People: Health Risks and Solutions: Factsheet No. 345*. [Online]. Available at: http://www.who.int/mediacentre/factsheets/fs345/en/index.html [Last accessed 23rd April 1013].

Wright, J., O'Flynn, G. and MacDonald, D. (2006). 'Being fit and looking healthy: young women's and men's constructions of health and fitness'. *Sex Roles*, 54 (9–10), 707–716.

Wrong, D. (2002). *Power: Its Forms, Bases and Uses*. (3rd ed.). London, UK: Transaction.

Wyness, M. (2009). 'Children representing children: participation and the problem of diversity in UK youth councils'. *Childhood*, 16 (4), 535–552.

———. (2012). 'Children's participation and intergenerational dialogue: bringing adults back into the analysis'. *Childhood*, doi:10.1177/0907568212459775.

Yeoh, P. L. (2009). 'Understanding health, culture and empowerment in a disability context'. *International Journal of Pharmaceutical and Healthcare Marketing*, 3 (2), 96–117.

Youdell, D. (2005). 'Sex – Gender – Sexuality: How sex, gender and sexuality constellations are constituted in secondary schools'. *Gender and Education*, 17 (3), 249–270.

Young, I. M. (1990). *Justice and the Politics of Difference*. Princeton, NJ: Princeton University Press.

Zaluar, A. (2001). 'Violence in Rio de Janeiro: Styles of leisure, drug use and trafficking'. *International Social Science Journal*, 53 (169), 369–378.

Zdun, S. (2008). 'Violence in street culture: cross-cultural comparison of youth groups and criminal gangs'. *Youth Development*, 119 (Autumn), 39–54.

Zimmerman, M. A. (1990). 'Taking aim on empowerment research: on the distinction between individual and psychological control'. *American Journal of Community Psychology*, 18 (1), 169–177.

———. (1995). 'Psychological empowerment: issues and illustrations'. *American Journal of Community Psychology*, 23 (5), 581–599.

Zimmerman, M. A. and Rappaport, J. (1988). 'Citizen participation, perceived control, and psychological empowerment'. *American Journal of Community Psychology*, 16 (5), 725–750.

Index

Page numbers in *italics* indicate figures or tables.

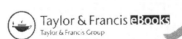